Laboratory Testing for Neurologic Disorders

Editor

A. ZARA HERSKOVITS

CLINICS IN LABORATORY MEDICINE

www.labmed.theclinics.com

Editor-in-Chief
MILENKO JOVAN TANASIJEVIC

September 2020 • Volume 40 • Number 3

ELSEVIER

1600 John F. Kennedy Boulevard • Suite 1800 • Philadelphia, Pennsylvania, 19103-2899

http://www.theclinics.com

CLINICS IN LABORATORY MEDICINE Volume 40, Number 3
September 2020 ISSN 0272-2712, ISBN-13: 978-0-323-76268-7

Editor: Katerina Heidhausen
Developmental Editor: Laura Fisher

Reprints. For copies of 100 or more, of articles in this publication, please contact the Commercial Reprints Department, Elsevier Inc., 360 Park Avenue South, New York, New York 10010-1710. Tel. 212-633-3874, Fax: 212-633-3820, E-mail: reprints@elsevier.com.

Clinics in Laboratory Medicine (ISSN 0272-2712) is published quarterly by Elsevier Inc., 360 Park Avenue South, New York, NY 10010-1710. Months of issue are March, June, September, and December. Business and Editorial offices: 1600 John F. Kennedy Blvd., Suite 1800, Philadelphia, PA 19103-2899. Periodicals postage paid at NewYork, NY and additional mailing offices. Subscription prices are $277.00 per year (US individuals), $571.00 per year (US institutions), $100.00 per year (US students), $349.00 per year (Canadian individuals), $693.00 per year (Canadian institutions), $100.00 per year (Canadian students), $404.00 per year (international individuals), $693.00 per year (international institutions), $185.00 (international students). Foreign air speed delivery is included in all Clinics subscription prices. All prices are subject to change without notice. POSTMASTER: Send address changes to *Clinics in Laboratory Medicine*, Elsevier Health Sciences Division, Subscription Customer Service, 3251 Riverport Lane, Maryland Heights, MO 63043. **Customer Service: 1-800-654-2452 (US). From outside of the US and Canada, call 1-314-447-8871. Fax: 1-314-447-8029. E-mail: journalscustomerservice-usa@elsevier.com (for print support) or journalsonlinesupport-usa@elsevier.com (for online support).**

Clinics in Laboratory Medicine is covered in *EMBASE/Exerpta Medica, MEDLINE/PubMed (Index Medicus), Cinahl, Current Contents/Clinical Medicine, BIOSIS* and *ISI/BIOMED.*

Contributors

EDITOR-IN-CHIEF

MILENKO JOVAN TANASIJEVIC, MD, MBA
Vice Chair for Clinical Pathology and Quality, Department of Pathology, Director of Clinical Laboratories, Brigham and Women's Hospital, Dana-Farber Cancer Institute, Associate Professor of Pathology, Harvard Medical School, Boston, Massachusetts

EDITOR

A. ZARA HERSKOVITS, MD, PhD
Department of Pathology, Co-Director of Clinical Chemistry, Beth Israel Deaconess Medical Center, Harvard Medical School, Boston, Massachusetts

AUTHORS

HESHAM ABBOUD, MD, PhD
Multiple Sclerosis and Neuroimmunology Program, Neurological Institute, University Hospitals Cleveland Medical Center, Case Western Reserve University School of Medicine, Cleveland, Ohio

JOHN F. BRANDSEMA, MD
Neuromuscular Section Head, Division of Neurology, Children's Hospital of Philadelphia, Assistant Professor of Clinical Neurology, Perelman School of Medicine, University of Pennsylvania, Philadelphia, Pennsylvania

BYRON CAUGHEY, PhD
Senior Investigator, Laboratory of Persistent Viral Diseases, Rocky Mountain Laboratories, National Institute for Allergy and Infectious Diseases, National Institutes of Health, Hamilton, Montana

ROBIN DAWN CLARK, MD
Division of Medical Genetics, Professor, Department of Pediatrics, Loma Linda University School of Medicine, Loma Linda, California

NATÁLIA DO CARMO FERREIRA, PhD
Postdoctoral Research Fellow, Laboratory of Persistent Viral Diseases, Rocky Mountain Laboratories, National Institute for Allergy and Infectious Diseases, National Institutes of Health, Hamilton, Montana

JAMIE C. FONG, MS, CGC
Department of Molecular and Human Genetics, Certified Genetic Counselor, Assistant Professor, Baylor College of Medicine, Houston, Texas

NEEL FOTEDAR, MD
Multiple Sclerosis and Neuroimmunology Program, Neurological Institute, University Hospitals Cleveland Medical Center, Case Western Reserve University School of Medicine, Cleveland, Ohio

NAVEEN GEORGE, DO, MHSA
Multiple Sclerosis and Neuroimmunology Program, Neurological Institute, University
Hospitals Cleveland Medical Center, Case Western Reserve University School of
Medicine, Cleveland, Ohio

JOSHUA F. GOLDSMITH, DO
Department of Pathology, Beth Israel Deaconess Medical Center, Harvard Medical
School, Boston, Massachusetts

BRIANNA N. GROSS, MS, LCGC
Neuromuscular Genetic Counselor, Children's Hospital of Philadelphia, Philadelphia,
Pennsylvania

YAEL K. HEHER, MD, MPH, FRCP(C)
Director, Quality & Patient Safety, Department of Pathology and Laboratory Medicine,
Beth Israel Deaconess Medical Center, Harvard Medical School, Boston, Massachusetts

A. ZARA HERSKOVITS, MD, PhD
Department of Pathology, Co-Director of Clinical Chemistry, Beth Israel Deaconess
Medical Center, Harvard Medical School, Boston, Massachusetts

GREGORY A. JICHA, MD, PhD
Department of Neurology, Sanders-Brown Center on Aging, University of Kentucky
College of Medicine, Lexington, Kentucky

LOREN J. JOSEPH, MD
Department of Pathology, Director of Molecular Pathology, Beth Israel Deaconess
Medical Center, Harvard Medical School, Boston, Massachusetts

SUSAN E. MATESANZ, MD
Neuromuscular Fellow, Children's Hospital of Philadelphia, Philadelphia, Pennsylvania

DAVID JOSHUA MICHELSON, MD
Assistant Professor, Division of Child Neurology, Department of Pediatrics, Loma Linda
University School of Medicine, Loma Linda, California

STANLEY J. NAIDES, MD
Director of Scientific Affairs, EUROIMMUN US, Mountain Lakes, New Jersey

JENNIFER ROGGENBUCK, MS, CGC
Division of Human Genetics, Department of Neurology, Certified Genetic Counselor,
Associate Clinical Professor, The Ohio State University, Columbus, Ohio

ISWARIYA VENKATARAMAN, PhD
Market Development Manager, Scientific Affairs, EUROIMMUN US, Mountain Lakes,
New Jersey

DONNA WILCOCK, PhD
Department of Physiology, Sanders-Brown Center on Aging, University of Kentucky
College of Medicine, Lexington, Kentucky

ZACHARY WINDER, BS
Department of Physiology, Sanders-Brown Center on Aging, University of Kentucky
College of Medicine, Lexington, Kentucky

Contents

Progress in medical genetics has changed the practice of medicine in general and child neurology in particular. A genetic diagnosis has become critically important in determining optimal management of many neurodevelopmental disorders, making genetic testing a routine consideration of patient care in outpatient and inpatient settings. Today's child neurologists should be familiar with various genetic testing modalities and their appropriate use. Molecular genetic testing of children with unexplained developmental delays and/or congenital anomalies has a 20% to 30% chance of identifying a causative etiology. Newer methods have made genetic testing more widely available and sensitive but also more likely to produce ambiguous results.

The need for etiological biomarkers for neurodegenerative diseases involving protein aggregation has prompted development of ultrasensitive cellular and cell-free assays based on the prion-like seeding capacity of such aggregates. Among them, prion RT-QuIC assays allow accurate antemortem Creutzfeldt-Jakob disease diagnosis using cerebrospinal fluid and nasal brushings. Analogous assays for synucleinopathies (e.g., Parkinson disease and dementia with Lewy bodies) provide unprecedented diagnostic sensitivity using cerebrospinal fluid. Biosensor cell and tau RT-QuIC assays can detect and discriminate tau aggregates associated with multiple tauopathies (e.g., Alzheimer disease and frontotemporal degeneration). An expanding panel of seed amplification assays should improve diagnostics and therapeutics development.

Amyotrophic lateral sclerosis (ALS) and frontotemporal dementia (FTD) are devastating neurodegenerative disorders that share clinical, pathologic, and genetic features. Persons and families affected by these conditions frequently question why they developed the disease, the expected disease course, treatment options, and the likelihood that family members will be affected. Genetic testing has the potential to answers these important questions. Despite the progress in gene discovery, the offer of genetic testing is not yet "standard of care" in ALS and FTD clinics. The authors review the current genetic landscape and present recommendations for the laboratory genetic evaluation of persons with these conditions.

This article focuses on current clinical laboratory testing to diagnose Alzheimer disease and monitor its progression throughout its disease course. Several clinically available tests focus on analysis of amyloid and tau levels in cerebrospinal fluid as well as autosomal dominant and risk factor genes. Although the current armament of clinical laboratory testing is limited by invasiveness of cerebrospinal fluid collection, rarity of autosomal dominant genetic mutations, and uncertainties of risk inherent in nonpenetrant genes, the field is poised to advance the clinical repertoire of laboratory diagnostic testing.

The recent discovery of several neuronal autoantibodies linked to neurologic syndromes that are fully or partially responsive to immunosuppressive therapy has revolutionized neuroimmunology and expanded the scope of classical paraneoplastic and antibody-related syndromes. A great deal of understanding of the techniques of neuronal antibody testing, the sensitivity and specificity of serum and cerebrospinal fluid sampling, and the value of the specific type and titer of each antibody is imperative. This article provides an overview of neuronal antibody and paraneoplastic panel testing with emphasis on how to differentiate clinically relevant from clinically irrelevant results and the downstream implications of those results.

Laboratory testing plays a critical role in the diagnosis and monitoring of patients with neurologic disorders. Although common tests are often performed in a central hospital laboratory, an increasing number of essential but esoteric tests are performed at reference laboratories or other outside health care facilities. In this article, we analyze recent trends in neurologic disease testing within the overall context of reference laboratory testing and discuss strategies to facilitate the provision of high-quality, cost-effective laboratory services.

Development of new diagnostic tests in a commercial laboratory for neurologic disorders is challenging. Development occurs in a highly regulated environment. Relevant research infrastructure may not be readily available in-house and may require outsourcing with additional management and costs. Clinically characterized specimens for validation of biomarkers for esoteric diseases may be difficult to acquire, and market size may be difficult to predict. More common diseases with heterogeneous subsets may require better clinical definition. Absence of guidelines may delay health provider acceptance of novel testing. Regulatory agency approval and categorization of tests affects validation requirements and impacts market acceptance and reimbursement.

Growing regulatory burdens, payment model changes, and increased complexity in laboratory medicine have contributed to an increased reliance on reference laboratories. Although reference laboratories often offer rapid, low cost, high quality testing, outsourcing laboratory tests can create quality and patient safety vulnerabilities particularly in the pre-analytic and post-analytic phases of the test cycle. Disconnects in governance, policy, and information technology between the reference laboratory and the referring provider conspire to increase risk. Laboratory leaders seeking to reduce risk and improve quality must ensure clear and collaborative oversight, monitor meaningful quality metrics, and integrate feedback from ordering providers.

Diagnostic genetic testing for spinal muscular atrophy is key in establishing early diagnosis for affected individuals. Prenatal carrier testing of parents with subsequent testing of the fetus for homozygous SMN1 gene deletion in those at risk of this autosomal recessive disorder as well as newborn screening can identify the vast majority of affected individuals before the onset of symptoms. Patients presenting symptomatically must be genetically confirmed as soon as possible because targeted treatments are now available that profoundly impact symptoms and improve quality of life.

Multiple sclerosis is one of the most common autoimmune diseases affecting the central nervous system. Current guidelines characterize multiple sclerosis and related conditions based on clinical, imaging, and body fluid markers. In this review, we describe how laboratory analysis of cerebrospinal fluid is currently performed and discuss new approaches under development for multiple sclerosis diagnostics.

CLINICS IN LABORATORY MEDICINE

SERIES OF RELATED INTEREST

Surgical Pathology Clinics
Available at: https://www.surgpath.theclinics.com/
Neurologic Clinics
Available at: https://www.neurologic.theclinics.com/

THE CLINICS ARE NOW AVAILABLE ONLINE!
Access your subscription at:
www.theclinics.com

Preface

Advances in Clinical Laboratory Testing for Neurologic Disorders

The number of cells in the human brain is thought to exceed the number of stars in our galaxy. Due to the tremendous scale and complexity of how brain cells interact, many factors can predispose patients to develop neurologic disease. Fortunately over the past ten years, there has been significant progress in our understanding of how to diagnose and treat patients with these complex disorders.

Identification of the genetic changes underlying several major neurologic diseases has been a significant driver of this progress. For example, diagnosis of spinal muscular atrophy (SMA) is multifaceted, characterized by mutations or deletions in the *SMN1* gene that can be accompanied with changes in the copy number of a second gene named *SMN2*. Together, these alterations determine the phenotypic severity of SMA. Unfortunately, the sequence similarity of these two homologous genes makes carrier screening and patient diagnosis challenging. Over the past five years, the Food and Drug Administration has approved two new treatments that may be curative. Selecting appropriate testing methodologies and correctly interpreting the results are of utmost importance for these patients and their families because accurately diagnosing this disease at an early age can profoundly impact clinical prognosis.

Another major genetic advance in this area is our understanding that amyotrophic lateral sclerosis and frontotemporal dementia can be linked with a hexanucleotide repeat expansion in the *C9ORF72* gene, and the length of this repeat is correlated with disease expression. Since the pathogenic allele exhibits somatic instability and can contain hundreds to thousands of guanine and cytosine repeats, the sequencing methodology and target tissue used for patient diagnosis must be carefully considered. Achieving accuracy and consistency in diagnostic methods is of paramount importance for counseling patients who may harbor this repeat expansion and for clinical trials targeting this gene.

Immunologic testing for neurologic diseases is another discipline that is growing at a rapid pace. The discovery of autoantibodies that cause encephalitis and paraneoplastic syndromes has been a major advance in terms of both diagnosis and treatment. Laboratory testing for these syndromes uses a range of analytic techniques, including enzyme-linked immunoassays, radioimmunoprecipitation assays, western blots, and cell-based immunofluorescence performed at different titers of patient serum. These tests are not trivial to develop and can be complex to interpret. Clear identification of pathogenic antibodies within the appropriate clinical context can direct cancer screening in patients with paraneoplastic syndromes and can also facilitate the selection of an appropriate treatment protocol for patients with encephalitis.

Another emerging frontier in laboratory testing for neurodegenerative disorders has stemmed from the discovery of how prion-mediated diseases are transmitted. It has been shown that conformationally altered prion protein can propagate disease by inducing structural change in the normal cellular form of this protein. This finding has

Clin Lab Med 40 (2020) ix–x
https://doi.org/10.1016/j.cll.2020.06.003
0272-2712/20/© 2020 Published by Elsevier Inc.

been applied to diagnostics using *ex vivo* amplification of pathogenic, misfolded proteins from clinical samples to detect abnormal prion protein. Similar analytic techniques have been applied to detect synuclein, beta-amyloid, and tau from patient samples, because conformationally altered forms of these proteins are found in Parkinson and Alzheimer disease. It remains to be seen whether these methodologies can be standardized, widely replicated, and incorporated into the workflow of immunoassay and nucleic acid tests that form the backbone of clinical laboratory testing.

It has been an honor and a wonderful learning experience to serve as guest editor for this issue of *Clinics in Laboratory Medicine*, and I greatly appreciate the expertise, time, and dedication of our authors as well as the editorial staff at Elsevier. I hope that this issue will be insightful for our readers by highlighting the progress that has been made in the area of neurologic disease testing and clarifying the work that remains ahead.

A. Zara Herskovits, MD, PhD
Department of Pathology
Beth Israel Deaconess Medical Center
Harvard Medical School
330 Brookline Avenue
Boston, MA 02215, USA

E-mail address:
aherskov@bidmc.harvard.edu

Optimizing Genetic Diagnosis of Neurodevelopmental Disorders in the Clinical Setting

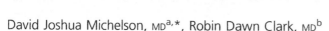

David Joshua Michelson, MD[a],*, Robin Dawn Clark, MD[b]

KEYWORDS

- Autism spectrum disorder, ASD • Genetic testing
- Global developmental delay, GDD • Intellectual disability, ID
- Multiple congenital anomalies, MCA • Neurodevelopmental disabilities, NDD
- Whole exome sequencing, WES • Whole genome sequencing, WGS

KEY POINTS

- Child neurologists play an important role in the genetic diagnosis of their patients.
- Molecular genetic testing of children with unexplained developmental delays and congenital anomalies has a 20% to 30% chance of identifying a causative etiology.
- Newer methods have made genetic testing more widely available and sensitive but also more likely to produce ambiguous results.
- Accurate interpretation of variants detected on genetic tests depends on the clarity and completeness of the phenotype and family history.
- Counseling before and after genetic testing helps families anticipate and understand the implications of positive, uncertain, and negative results.

INTRODUCTION

Neurodevelopmental disabilities (NDDs) affect 2% to 3% of children and require large investments of medical and supportive care from families, clinicians, and society. Monitoring child development and identifying NDDs allows for the initiation of supportive therapies at an early age, when they are the most likely to improve outcomes. Finding a specific cause for NDDs has the potential to lead to more effective early intervention, causal treatments, anticipation of comorbidities, and counseling for

[a] Division of Child Neurology, Department of Pediatrics, Loma Linda University School of Medicine, Coleman Pavilion Room A, 1175 Campus Street, Loma Linda, CA 92354, USA;
[b] Division of Medical Genetics, Department of Pediatrics, Loma Linda University School of Medicine, Coleman Pavilion Room A, 1175 Campus Street, Loma Linda, CA 92354, USA
* Corresponding author.
E-mail address: dmichels@llu.edu

Clin Lab Med 40 (2020) 231–256
https://doi.org/10.1016/j.cll.2020.05.001
0272-2712/20/© 2020 Elsevier Inc. All rights reserved.

labmed.theclinics.com

parents about prognosis and recurrence risk. NDDs can be the result of prenatal, perinatal, and postnatal injuries and diseases, but it is estimated that at least 20% to 30%
of cases have a genetic cause. Multiple congenital anomalies (MCAs) in the context of
NDDs can help narrow the differential diagnosis and therefore deserve special consideration in the diagnostic evaluation. The diagnostic yield for genetic disorders in patients with NDDs is higher in those with MCAs. Main categories of neurologic
impairment and their diagnostic criteria are reviewed later. Recommendations and
strategies for genetic testing based on patterns of clinical findings are elaborated later
(Clinical Approach).

Global Developmental Delay

A child with global developmental delay (GDD) shows significant delay (falling more
than 2 standard deviations behind age-related norms) in 2 or more aspects of development.[1] These aspects include the following:

- Gross motor movements and fine motor movements
- Cognitive function including reasoning, problem-solving, memory, and learning
- Receptive and expressive language
- Socialization and reciprocation
- Adaptive functioning such as toileting, dressing, and grooming

An estimated 5% of children younger than 5 years in the United States and Canada are
believed to meet criteria for the diagnosis of GDD, although only 3% will eventually meet
criteria for the more specific diagnosis of intellectual disability (ID) when they are older
than 7 years, when intelligence quotient (IQ) testing is considered sufficiently reliable.

Intellectual Disability

ID is defined by the fifth edition of the Diagnostic and Statistical Manual of Mental Disorder (DSM-5) as a neurodevelopmental disorder that begins in early childhood and
causes difficulties with conceptual, practical, and social aspects of living due to deficits in perceptual and quantitative reasoning, verbal comprehension, abstract
thought, comprehending instructions and rules, memory, problem-solving, and
learning from experience.[2] ID can be stratified by severity into 4 levels (**Fig. 1**). There

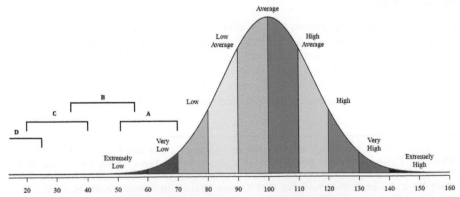

Fig. 1. Subdivision of intellectual disability (ID) into categories, based on intelligence quotient (IQ). (A) Mild ID with IQ between 50 and 70; (B) moderate ID with IQ between 35–
55, (C) severe ID with IQ between 20–40, and (D) profound ID with IQ less than 25. These
are overlapping categories not defined strictly by IQ. The likelihood of single gene disorder
increases and the IQ decreases.

is an inverse correlation between IQ and the likelihood of a positive genetic diagnosis. Genetic tests, such as chromosome microarray and genetic or genomic sequencing, have a higher yield in patients with severe or profound ID, whereas those with borderline or mild ID are less likely to have positive results.

About 85% of individuals with ID have mild ID, with an IQ between 50 and 70, are typically able to learn and retain information related to performing activities of daily living, perform well in social situations, and require minimal assistance other than when making complex decisions. Moderate ID is seen in about 10% of those with ID, with IQ scores ranging from 35 to 55, more limited ability to learn skills related to personal health and safety, and greater need for assistance in their daily lives. Severe ID accounts for 3.5% of all ID and is associated with IQ scores of 20 to 35; difficulty learning more than simple routines and basic self-care skills; restricted receptive and expressive language abilities; and the need for more direct supervision in performing everyday activities, behaving appropriately in social settings, and maintaining health and safety. Individuals with profound ID, making up 1.5% of all cases of ID, have IQ scores less than 20 and exhibit extremely limited ability to learn self-care skills and require around-the-clock assistance with activities of daily living. Although mild or moderate ID may only become recognizable in school-age children as they struggle with academic performance, children with moderate to severe ID often suffer from other medical issues and are recognized in the first 2 years of life.[3]

Autism Spectrum Disorders

Children with autism spectrum disorders (ASDs) show characteristic impairments in social communication, repetitive and restricted behaviors, and unusual sensory sensitivities and interests. The prevalence of ASDs has been estimated to be as high as 1 in 36 children, with a male to female ratio of about 4 to 5:1.[4] The DSM-5 collapses terms used previously—autistic disorder, Asperger disorder, and pervasive developmental disorder-not otherwise specified—into a single umbrella category.[5] People with ASDs are more likely than the general population to have other neuropsychological disabilities, including receptive and expressive language impairments, specific learning disabilities, and ID, and to suffer from other neurologic comorbidities including psychiatric disorders and epilepsy.[6] Women with autism, being the less commonly affected sex, have a higher threshold for this diagnosis and are more likely to have an identifiable genetic cause. Characterizing autism into subcategories (autism and macrocephaly, epilepsy, developmental regression, borderline autistic phenotype in the parents, those with older paternal age, etc.) may provide useful designations for specific testing strategies.

Congenital Anomalies

Congenital anomalies (CA) may be major or minor.[7] Major CA are those that have significant medical, social, or cosmetic consequences and typically require medical intervention, such as an absent kidney or cleft palate. Minor CA are those that have little or no impact on the individual and need no intervention, such as a single palmar crease or low hairline.

Most major CA occur in isolation but can be accompanied by additional minor anomalies, whereas about 25% of major CA are multiple (MCA). Multiple anomalies that result from a single disrupting influence or mechanical factor are referred to as a sequence. An example is the holoprosencephaly sequence, in which the absence of midline brain structures leads to lack of development of midline facial features, which can cause hypotelorism, cleft lip, single nostril, single central maxillary incisor, loss of midline labial frenulum, and anosmia, some of which are microforms that can be seen in parents, who might only come to medical attention after having a severely affected child. A pattern of MCAs that is thought to have a single underlying pathogenetic cause, whether genetic or environmental, is referred to as a syndrome. Examples include Down syndrome, due to trisomy 21, and congenital cytomegalovirus (CMV) syndrome, due to maternal infection with CMV.

A pattern of MCAs without a known cause that occur together more often than expected by chance alone is referred to as an association. Previously known as the CHARGE association of Coloboma, Heart defect, choanal Atresia, Retardation of growth and/or development, and Genetourinary and Ear anomalies, this pattern of anomalies has been redefined as a syndrome, as most cases have heterozygous mutations of *CHD7*. The VACTERL association of Vertebral, Anal, Cardiac, Trachea-Esophageal fistula, Renal, and Limb defects remains unexplained by any known genetic or environmental factor.

Overall, about 40% of CA are thought to have a direct genetic cause, which could be chromosomal, multifactorial, or single gene disorder. Numerical and structural chromosomal abnormalities (trisomies and monosomies such as Down syndrome and Turner syndrome) include contiguous gene syndromes: duplication or deletion such as the contiguous gene deletion syndrome of 22q11.2 or velocardiofacial syndrome. Together these make up about 10% of cases of MCAs and are usually recognized clinically by their distinctive patterns. About 5% to 10% of CA are thought to be due to identifiable environmental and maternal causes such as teratogenic agents (alcohol), malnutrition, drug and toxin exposure, and maternal infection and disease.

CA can be subcategorized according to developmental mechanism. The first 2 categories describe inherently abnormal morphogenesis, with a higher likelihood of genetic cause. The last 2 categories describe external factors that derange otherwise normal development, with a lower likelihood of genetic causation.

- A *malformation* is a disturbance of the initial formation of an organ or body region, leading to an abnormal, incomplete, or absent structure. Examples include anencephaly and spina bifida.
- A *dysplasia* refers to the abnormal formation of organ derived from a single tissue type such as skin, brain, or bone. Examples include ectodermal dysplasia or achondroplasia.
- A *disruption* is a destructive process that affects an organ or body region that was otherwise developing normally. Examples include amniotic band disruption sequence and intrauterine cerebral infarction.
- A *deformation* results from abnormal mechanical forces that change the shape of an otherwise normal developing body part. Examples include oligohydramnios after prematurely ruptured membranes leading to Potter sequence (distinctive facial findings, lung hypoplasia, and clubfoot).

Diagnostic Genetic Testing

A substantial amount of research on etiologic testing of NDDs has focused on patients from these 3 categories: GDD, ASD, and ID. About 70% of patients with ASD will also meet criteria for GDD/ID, and many chromosomal anomalies and single gene disorders have variable phenotypic expression that can include ASD, GDD/ID, or both. Similarly, patients with MCAs are often included in retrospective studies of diagnostic yield of screening genetic tests. A detailed approach offers better phenotyping information through careful history taking, including family history, and thorough examination of the patient and, when appropriate, the parents.

A positive genetic test result that establishes a new or newly confirmed clinical diagnosis improves a clinician's ability to provide the following:

- Recurrence risk and genetic counseling to the family
- Referrals to therapy programs, support and advocacy groups, and research projects
- Specific treatments based on the pathophysiology of the condition
- Tailored referrals, testing, and follow-up based on associated comorbidities such as vision loss, hearing loss, epilepsy, hyperphagia, hypogonadism, immune deficiency, or cardiac involvement
- Accurate information about long-term prognosis, longevity, and fertility

It is estimated that 30% to 40% of NDD have a genetic cause, although not all are detectable with current techniques. The most commonly identified genetic errors are copy number variants (CNVs) and other chromosomal anomalies.[8] The most recent consensus from the American College of Medical Genetics, published in 2010, recommended the use of a chromosomal microarray (CMA) as the first tier of genomic analysis for patients presenting with unexplained GDD/ID or CMA.[9] The next step after microarray, if microarray is negative, is less clear. Whole exome sequencing (WES) testing may become sufficiently cost-effective to become a first or second tier test. At present, fragile X testing is still considered an appropriate next test for men with severe NDD, women with any degree of NDD, or anyone with an X-linked family history, although the presence of microcephaly or other major CA would argue against fragile X syndrome as a single etiologic cause. It should be remembered that some individuals with NDD have more than one diagnosis (genetic or environmental) underlying their disability, which argues for a broader testing approach, especially when a positive genetic test does not adequately explain the patient's phenotype.

TYPES OF GENETIC TESTS

Genetic testing options range in scope from the narrowest, single gene approach, to the broadest, whole genome test. Genetic defects also range in size from a single nucleotide polymorphism to large CNVs millions of bases in size that include hundreds of individual genes (**Fig. 2**). Matching the right test to the right patient requires an appropriate understanding of what type of pathologic changes each test can and cannot detect.

Chromosome Analysis: a Low-Resolution Whole Genome Analysis

A G-banded karyotype is a photographic representation of the entire set of 46 chromosomes, captured in metaphase during cell division, which has been visually inspected for numeric and large structural changes such as deletions, duplications, rearrangements, and inversions (**Fig. 3**). The chromosomes, and smaller regions within them, are distinguished by the patterns of light and dark bands that appear following trypsin digestion and Giemsa staining. Transcriptionally active (euchromatic) regions are in a less condensed configuration, with proteins that are more accessible to trypsin for digestion. The Giemsa stain preferentially binds to the proteins associated with the less active (heterochromatic) regions that are in a more condensed configuration.[10] Chromosome analysis done using a blood sample routinely stimulates T-cell lymphocytes to divide ex-vivo using phytohemagglutinin. When chromosome analysis fails, it may be due to insufficient or abnormal T cells, such as in 22q11.2 deletion syndrome. Other tissues, such as fibroblast culture from skin biopsies, can be used for chromosome analysis. A helpful online resource for chromosome morphology is available at

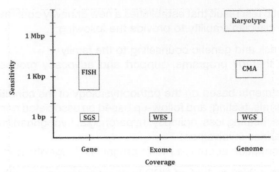

Fig. 2. Relative coverage and sensitivity of clinical genetic tests. CMA, chromosomal micro-array, FISH, fluorescence in situ hybridization, SGS, single gene sequencing, WES, whole exome sequencing, WGS, whole genome sequencing. In the cartographic metaphor of genetic testing, a "Google Earth" or satellite view of the genome is offered by the karyotype, which produces an overall assessment of the genome at low resolution. The "Google Street view" map is provided by exome sequencing, which looks at the genome from one point of view, prioritizing the regions that produce gene products.

the University of Washington: http://www.pathology.washington.edu/research/cytopages/idiograms/human/.

High-resolution karyotyping provides the highest possible resolution (750–800 bands), and yet even this technique is unable to detect changes affecting fewer than several millions of base pairs (Mb). Chromosome analysis has largely been supplanted by more sensitive techniques that detect deletions and duplications at a far smaller scale. Banding is not uniformly distributed and it is particularly difficult to see changes in some regions, such that karyotyping can fail to detect copy number changes as large as 10 Mb. Furthermore, the subjective nature of the visual inspection involved in karyotype analysis makes the test highly prone to interrater variability in detection of abnormalities.

Overall, chromosome analysis has a yield of about 3% when applied to cases of developmental disability of unknown cause.[11] The American College of Medical Genetics and Genomics has recommended that karyotyping be used in cases where a large chromosomal rearrangement is suspected (eg, trisomy of chromosome 21 in Down syndrome) or when the family history suggests that a parent may carry a balanced translocation (eg, recurrent pregnancy loss or miscarriage).[9] With laboratories performing fewer karyotypes, however, expertise in interpretation seems to be fading.[12]

Chromosomal Microarray: a Higher Resolution Whole Genome Analysis

CMA has replaced conventional chromosome analysis as a first-line test. It is more sensitive for the detection of microdeletions and microduplications, CNVs composed of thousands rather than millions of base pairs. In studies of developmental disabilities, CMA analyses find diagnostic CNVs in 5% to 10% in subjects with nonsyndromic autism and in 20% to 25% of subjects with moderate to severe ID accompanied by dysmorphic facial features or congenital malformations.[13] Unlike conventional chromosome analysis, CMA cannot detect balanced or structural chromosome rearrangements such as inversions, rings, and translocations. However, such structural chromosome changes are rare: present in 1 in 1000 in the general population and in less than 1% of the disabled population.

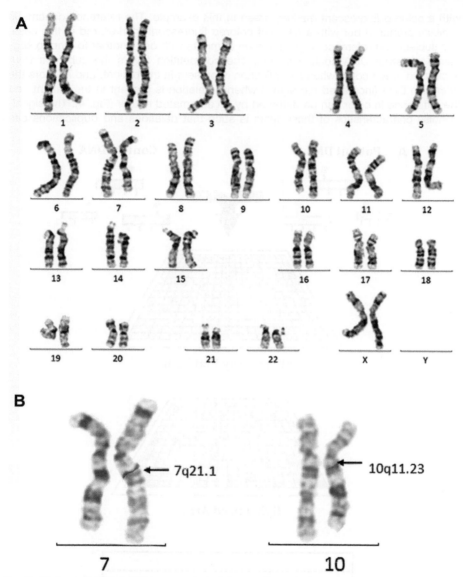

Fig. 3. High-resolution karyotype analysis (*A*) revealing a balanced translocation between 7q21.1 and 10q11.23 (*B*) detected in a woman pursuing in vitro fertilization following 2 consecutive miscarriages. (*From* Tšuiko O, Dmitrijeva T, Kask K, et al. Detection of a balanced translocation carrier through trophectoderm biopsy analysis: a case report. Mol Cytogenet. 2019;12:28. The figure is distributed under the terms of the Creative Commons Attribution 4.0 International License (http://creativecommons.org/licenses/by/4.0/). This version of the figure has been modified to add color.)

Two techniques are in widespread use: array comparative genomic hybridization (aCGH) and single nucleotide polymorphism (SNP) arrays. aCGH compares a subject's genome to a reference standard. The subject's DNA is separated into single strands, digested into small segments using restriction enzymes, and then labeled with a colored fluorescent marker, green in this example. The reference genome is similarly prepared but with a different colored fluorescent marker, red in this case. The subject and reference segments then compete with one another to bind to segments of target DNA coating a chip. The competition favors the subject's DNA (increased green color) when a duplication is present in the patient, and it favors the reference DNA (increased red signal) when a deletion is present in the patient and the difference in color can be detected by an automated reader (**Fig. 4**). The signal-to-noise characteristics of these tests is such that deletions and duplications can

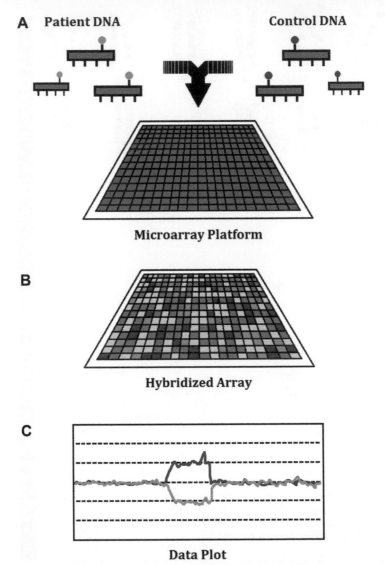

Fig. 4. Array comparative genomic hybridization (aCGH) labels digested segments of single-stranded DNA from a patient (*green*) and a reference control (*red*) fluorescence (*A*), allows competitive hybridization on an array platform of complimentary reference DNA (*B*), and then uses automated analysis of the results to create a data plot (*C*) that shows any areas of copy number variation.

reliably be detected in a region covered by as few as 3 to 6 oligonucleotides, which may represent a single exon of a gene.[14]

Individual genomes contain, on average, 4 to 5 million single nucleotide variations from the reference human genome. Variants of this nature that occur in more than 1% of the population are called SNP or "snip". An SNP array digests and labels the subject's DNA into oligonucleotides as small as 20 base pairs and then creates a genotype by probing for SNPs using either single-base extension reactions (Illumina methodology) or hybridization (Affymetrix methodology).

SNP arrays detect copy number changes but also identify copy-neutral changes such as regions of homozygosity (ROH, or absence of heterozygosity), an indicator of uniparental disomy (when both copies of a chromosome come from just one parent) and parental consanguinity (when both parents share a common ancestry). SNP arrays are also more sensitive than aCGH for low-level mosaicism. SNPs are not evenly distributed throughout the genome, such that SNP arrays are insensitive to copy number changes in some regions. Providers should be aware that SNP microarrays may detect incestuous relationships that are unacknowledged, creating a counseling dilemma.

CMA methods in general struggle to detect low copy repeat (LCR) sequences, highly repetitive sequences, and highly homologous sequences such as pseudogenes. Laboratories can use various combinations of comparative hybridization and SNP analysis to achieve optimal sensitivity for clinically relevant CNV and ROH.[15]

Microarray Nomenclature

Chromosome abnormalities identified by microarray are described using the International System for Human Cytogenomic Nomenclature, which is regularly updated, most recently in 2016. Normal microarray results indicate that the chromosome pairs are present in 2 copies. Normal female and male results are reported, respectively, as arr(1–22,X)x2 or arr(1–22)x2,(X,Y)x1. Abnormal microarray results are expressed in terms of the genomic position of the copy number change within a specific version of the genomic map. More than 3 billion nucleotides in the human genome have been assembled into a map, but this map continues to be refined and updated with new revisions. Not surprisingly, reference points change with different versions. Microarray results reference the version of the human genome map that was used to generate the coordinates that are being reported, usually in hard brackets: [hg19] for human genome map 19 or [GRCh38/hg38] for Genome Reference Consortium Human Genome Build map 38. The map version is followed by the chromosome bands for the region involved. This is followed by two 9-digit (usually) numbers, separated by a dash, and enclosed within a set of parentheses, followed by the times symbol ("x") and the number of copies identified. For example, arr[hg19]4q32.2q35.1(163146681–183022312) x1 describes a deletion of the long arm of chromosome 4 from band 4q32.2 to 4q35.1, using coordinates from Human Genome map 19. The 9-digit numbers refer to the genomic positions of the nucleotides that mark the start and stop positions of the CNV. The length of the CNV can be determined by subtracting the smaller parenthetic number from the larger one: in this case, the deletion size is 19.8 Mb (1 Mb = 1,000,000 nucleotides). By inputting the map version, chromosome number, and genomic coordinates into a genome browser, a list of genes within the CNV can be obtained. The genome browser maintained by the University of California at Santa Cruz is a useful resource: https://genome.ucsc.edu/.

Fluorescence In Situ Hybridization

Fluorescence in situ hybridization (FISH) analysis determines whether a specific DNA sequence is present within a genetic sample, using a short, single-stranded DNA probe with a fluorescent label that is complementary to the region of interest (**Fig. 5**). FISH studies can be performed in dividing cells in metaphase or in fixed tissues in interphase and the latter can be performed quickly because no cell culture is needed. FISH is a sensitive test when a particular deletion is suspected, when parental testing is recommended after identifying a deletion in a child, or when mosaicism is under consideration. FISH is less useful for duplications because 2 positive signals may seem as one when the signals are adjacent to one another; which is why interphase preparations are often preferred. FISH is useful because it is relatively quick and less expensive than other options when a recurrent CNV is suspected and deletion and/or duplication of a single gene region contributes substantially to the cause (such as in 22q11.2 deletion [DiGeorge or velocardiofacial syndrome]). FISH is not useful when the phenotype is nonspecific. A microarray is a better test in that situation.

Methylation Testing

Southern blot analysis of DNA fragment length using restriction enzymes that only cut unmethylated sequences are used to detect genetic disorders associated with imprinted genes. The 15q11.13 region contains multiple genes that are imprinted when they are passed on by the mother and just one gene, *UBE3A*, which is imprinted when it is passed on by the father. When methylation-dependent digestion is performed, paternally derived copies of this region will be cut into smaller fragments than maternally derived copies. Angelman syndrome (AS) is due to loss of function of *UBE3A* in about 90% of cases.[16] An abnormal Southern blot using this methylation-dependent digestion that shows only small fragments suggests absence of the maternal allele, which can be caused by deletion within the maternal 15q11.13 region (seen in 65%–75% of patients with AS), uniparental disomy of the paternal chromosome 15 (3%–7% of cases of AS), or an imprinting defect (3% of cases).

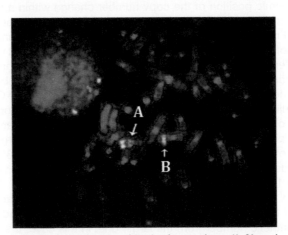

Fig. 5. Fluorescence in situ hybridization (FISH) of interphase (*left*) and metaphase (*right*) chromosomes illustrating a single hybridization signal (labeled *red*) for the target region on 7q11.23, within the Williams Syndrome Critical Region, as well as 2 hybridization signals for the control region (labeled *green*) on distal chromosome 7q. After hybridization, one normal chromosome shows a red signal next to a green control signal (A), but the deleted chromosome 7 shows only the control signal, indicating deletion of the target 7q11.23 region (B). (*From* Souza, DH, Moretti-Ferreira D, Rugolo, LMSS. Fluorescent in situ hybridization (FISH) as a diagnostic tool for Williams-Beuren syndrome. Gen Mol Bio. 2007;30(1):18; with permission.)

Fragile X syndrome is usually associated with the presence of more than 200 CGG trinucleotide repeats in the 5′ untranslated region of the *FMR1* gene. Subjects with between 55 and 200 repeats are at some risk of early ovarian failure and neurodegenerative disease later in life but are considered premutation carriers, at risk for producing offspring with a repeat sequence expanded into the full mutation range. Full mutations cause hypermethylation of *FMR1*, which can be detected as larger restriction fragments on Southern blot testing using methylation-inactivated restriction enzyme digestion. In the last few years, however, polymerase chain reaction (PCR) testing of this region has improved to the point that expansion lengths can be measured reliably.[17] Microarray techniques are being adapted to allow detection of abnormal methylation patterns in patients with developmental disabilities.[18]

Genetic and Genomic Sequencing

Although massively parallel gene sequencing has become the more cost-effective and rapid sequencing option, DNA was originally sequenced in a stepwise fashion, one base pair at a time, using one of several older techniques. The Sanger technique, first introduced in 1977, brought about a revolution in medicine, allowing clinicians to diagnose genetic disease and researchers to investigate specific genotype-phenotype correlations. Sanger sequencing was used to generate most of the data for the Human Genome Project, a massive 13-year, $3 billion effort to produce the first complete map of the human genome.

Sanger Sequencing: Low-Volume, High-Cost, Focused Genetic Testing with Highest Accuracy

The process begins with a DNA sample that is denatured into 2 single strands. Then the target areas are bound by a specifically designed primer sequence to initiate further replication. This short region of double-stranded DNA serves as the base for DNA polymerase, which extends the primer and completes the missing sequence using the intact strand as the template. The process is carried out in the presence of both normal and sequence terminating nucleotides that stop any further complementary strand extension once they are incorporated. These defective nucleotides are fluorescently labeled with colors that indicate their nucleotide type. The process is repeated thousands of times, resulting in complementary DNA strands of differing lengths, each ending with a labeled nucleotide at their 3′ end. The mix of strands is run through capillary electrophoresis so that the color at the end of each segment is read by a laser and photodetector in sequence, from smallest (moving fastest through the gel) to largest (**Fig. 6**), establishing the order of the nucleotides in the completed sequence. The technique is time consuming and costly, but it is still considered the gold standard for accurate genetic testing. Sanger sequencing continues to have clinical application for targeted testing and single gene analysis.

Next-Generation Sequencing: High-Volume, Low-Cost, Hypothesis-Free Genomic Testing

Since 2004, the emergence of next-generation sequencing (NGS) techniques has brought about a second revolution making genetic testing in any of hundreds or thousands of genes available and affordable for the general medical community. Instead of pursuing one genetic test at a time, the economics of NGS favor a broader, hypothesis-free, genomic approach to testing. This approach casts a wide net, which may be advantageous in detecting new genes and novel associations, but it also generates data indiscriminately, returning variants that cannot be interpreted due to lack

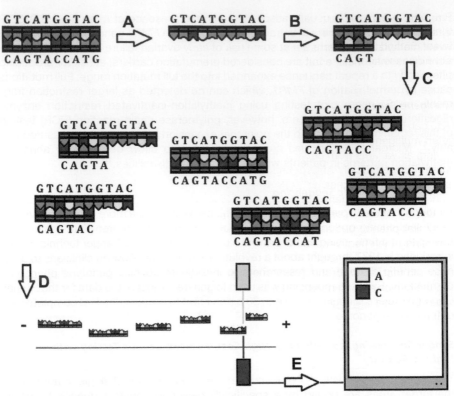

Fig. 6. Sanger sequencing technique, starting with a sample of DNA that is then (A) denatured into a single strand and (B) joined to a primer for DNA polymerase to (C) extend using both normal nucleotides and color-labeled dideoxyribonucleic acids that terminate the polymerase reaction, resulting in fragments of varying length that can be (D) run through electrophoresis toward a laser and photodetector that (E) transmits to a computer the color of each 3′ terminal nucleotide in order from shortest to longest fragment.

of sufficient clinical data. These variants of unknown significance (VUS) add to the difficulties of interpreting results for patients.

The NGS technique uses massively parallel processing of millions of small DNA fragments to produce partial sequences (reads) that can be reassembled using analytical tools into a full sequence.

There have been several competing NGS techniques, developed by rival companies over the years, but currently the Illumina platform for NGS dominates the market. In this array-based method, DNA is fragmented into segments of about 250 base pairs, denatured into single strands, which are then bound on both ends by adapter sequences. For tests done on regions of interest, test fragments are selectively hybridized to DNA probes referred to as primers or bait. The fragments are bound to a glass slide, amplified numerous times into bundles, and then elongated by DNA polymerase using nucleotides that are modified so that they emit a base-specific flash of color as they are bound. The sequencing device records each flash, collecting millions of pieces of sequence information from across the slide simultaneously. This fragmented information is recombined into a complete sequence of the whole DNA sample by aligning overlapping regions (**Fig. 7**). Because the human genome contains regions of repetitive DNA that are longer than the fragment length used by NGS platforms, the reassembly process for these regions is prone to error. Numerous NGS methods that reveal methylation patterns in DNA are the subject of active research. With time, these techniques may yield another layer of genetic information that is associated with disease.[19]

Multigene Panels

NGS can be applied to any number of genes with a common phenotype to provide targeted multigene panels. This approach has its advantages over more genome-wide testing, as variants from genes not matching the patient's phenotype will not be evaluated. For genetically heterogeneous conditions such as nonsyndromic ID or ASD, panels can be designed to perform enriched sampling of some or all of the more than one thousand genes previously linked to these conditions.[20] However, panels curated by different commercial laboratories differ in the choice and number of genes for similar phenotypes and also in their detection rates. There have been no studies comparing the effectiveness of different gene panels in NDDs. Without a consensus as to which genes to include, choosing the best gene panel may be a hit or miss experience. In fact, some of the genes in these panels may not add to the detection rate, and the cynics among us suggest that some genes may be added for marketing purposes because larger gene panels seem to promise a higher diagnostic yield. The use

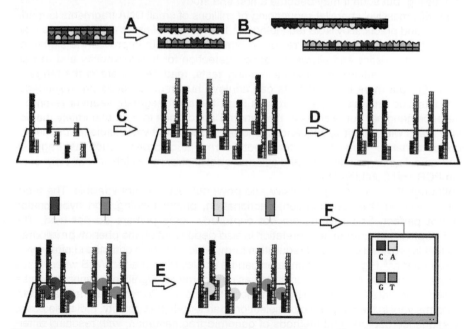

Fig. 7. In next-generation sequencing (NGS) done on platforms offered by Illumina, a DNA sample is (A, B) denatured, fragmented, and bound on both ends by adaptors (purple and orange). The fragments are then bound by complimentary adaptors on a matrix where (C) multiple copies of these fragments are copied and (D) separated into like bundles through multiple rounds of PCR bridge amplification, resulting in short single-strand bundles anchored at one end. Individual colonies are then (E) polymerized using nucleotides, which emit a base-specific color as they bind, reflecting the sequence of the fragment. The light is collected by cameras and (F) recorded by a computer as fragment sequences that can then be reconstructed using areas of overlap into a complete sequence of the original DNA.

of gene panels that focus on known genes forecloses on the potential for discovering novel genetic associations, and the evidence is growing for a genomic approach rather than a preselected gene panel.

Whole Exome Sequencing

The human genome contains some 22 thousand genes, with just 1% to 2% of the total 3.2 billion base pairs making up the protein-encoding exonic regions, or exome. Another 26% of genomic DNA makes up the intronic regions between exons and the remaining 72% to 73% is made up of intragenic, noncoding DNA.[21] The regulatory role played by introns and noncoding segments (promoters, enhancers, and other transcriptional modifiers such as cis-acting RNAs) is increasingly understood, which makes interpretation of variants in noncoding regions important but challenging.[22] Further gene regulation is applied by epigenetic elements such as chromatin marks, methylation, and acetylation of histone proteins, which will undoubtedly be the object of future advances in genetic testing.

The utility of WES as a first tier test has been supported by a recent meta-analysis of 30 studies, which found a diagnostic yield of 36% in children with unexplained NDDs and 53% in children with NDD associated with any additional clinical findings.[23] At this time, WES or clinical exome sequencing are used primarily to study subjects with suspected genetic disease in whom one or more conventional genetic tests have been unrevealing, but soon it may become a first line study.

In WES, massively parallel sequencing of millions of small DNA fragments is made possible and practical by NGS technology.[24] The number of times a nucleotide is read defines the read-depth for that region. A higher read-depth improves the signal-to-noise characteristics and allows increased detection for heterozygosity and mosaicism. For most regions, on broad screening tests, read depths are in the range of 50 to 100, but more targeted tests can achieve hundreds of reads per nucleotide. Computerized analysis maps the results from the short segment sequences onto a reference genome. Some areas of the genome are difficult to read accurately, particularly areas with repetitive sequences, and thus NGS is not yet reliable for the detection of dynamic mutations in trinucleotide repeat disorders, such as fragile X syndrome, Huntington disease, and spinocerebellar atrophy, which are still diagnosed with PCR and Southern blotting.

Although WES is a comprehensive and powerful test, it is not infallible. The techniques used in DNA denaturation, fractionation, primer binding, and hybridization are not perfect. Some exons are not captured. Some primers do not bind. The read-depth is not uniform. Interpretation is also dependent on the phenotype information that is provided on the test requisition form, which can be a critical and often overlooked factor.[25] Higher detection rates can be achieved with a trio WES when tissue samples from both parents are included as comparators. Significant variants may be missed if they interfere with the hybridization of primers.[22] Commercially available test platforms vary in their target region selection, bait length, bait density, molecules used for sequence capture, and methods of genomic fragmentation, with resulting differences in target enrichment efficiency, coverage of untranslated regions, sensitivity for single nucleotide variants (SNVs), short insertions or deletions (indels), medically interesting mutations, and homozygous SNVs.[26] NGS can detect some CNVs as small as 1000 base pairs, with sensitivities greater than 95% for some algorithms, although high false detection rates remain problematic.[27] Interpretation depends on accurate and complete annotation of variants in various populations around the world. Unfortunately, people of color and populations from developing countries have historically been underrepresented in major genomic databases.[28] A diagnosis may be made simply by requesting reinterpretation of negative WES data after 1 to 2 years, a laboratory service that must be requested but is often available at no additional charge.

Whole Genome Sequencing

Whole genome sequencing (WGS) covers the entire genome, both coding and noncoding regions, and produces a more complete dataset of genomic variants. The diagnostic yield for WGS exceeds WES.[29] The main impediments to the wider application of WGS are practical ones involving cost and data management. As these challenges are overcome, we expect that WGS will overtake WES as the preferred platform for genomic analysis.

Although the sequencing costs of performing WGS are approaching those of WES, more than 100 times more data are produced by WGS, with a much larger number of variants. This creates challenges in storing, managing, and analyzing WGS results. Noncoding regions of the genome tolerate more variability than exons, and variants from noncoding regions are less easily interpreted for pathogenicity.[30,31] Disease-causing mutations have historically been found more often within exons, although this may reflect a sampling bias.[32] Recent studies from WGS are beginning to identify sequence conservation and functionally deleterious variants within noncoding regions.[33] NGS can sequence the breakpoints involved in seemingly balanced chromosomal rearrangements identified by CMA, elucidating the cause of pathology in symptomatic patients.[34] Methods are being developed to allow copy-neutral rearrangements, such as inversions, to be detected by WGS.[35]

Mitochondrial DNA Sequencing

NGS has been successfully adapted to diagnose mitochondrial disease by enhanced coverage of the more than 1400 nuclear genes that are known to be directly or indirectly involved in mitochondrial function and by sequencing the maternally-inherited mitochondrial genome (mtDNA). This dual genome approach using NGS is the recommended first-line test for the genetic evaluation of patients suspected to have a mitochondrial disorder.[36] Lymphocytes may have low levels of heteroplasmy, which limits test sensitivity in blood samples. Choosing tissues with a higher mtDNA content than blood, such renal epithelial cells as collected from urine, or tissues that are clinically affected, such as the liver or muscle, offers greater test sensitivity. With the use of novel analytical techniques, NGS-based testing detects levels of mtDNA heteroplasmy as low as 0.2%.[37]

Third-Generation Sequencing

The third-generation sequencing methods address some of the common shortfalls of NGS. TGS methods use a single DNA molecule and avoid the need for amplification and error-prone PCR in GC-rich regions. TGS can sequence long DNA fragments decreasing the need for fragmentation and some of the challenges of reassembly. The first TGS technology, called single-molecule real-time (SMRT) sequencing, was introduced in 2011 by Pacific Biosciences. An SMRT cell contains 150,000 zeptoliter $(10^{-21}L)$ wells, each holding a single, immobilized molecule of DNA polymerase. A template single-strand DNA molecule is coupled with the DNA polymerase and a complimentary strand is synthesized using fluorescently labeled nucleotides. The emitted color is continuously recorded by CCD cameras, providing sequence information in real time. The use of circularized templates allows this system to produce longer and more accurate reads.[38]

CLINICAL APPROACH

Genetic testing in a child with NDD or CMA is more effective when the clinical evaluation begins with a thorough medical history, including pregnancy, birth, and developmental histories, a 3-generation family history, and culminates in a detailed physical examination. This process documents the phenotype, which not only improves the chance of a clinical diagnosis but also guides the selection of the most appropriate genetic test strategy. The quality of the clinical information communicated to the laboratory on the test requisition form also enhances the interpretation of genetic results. It may be worthwhile to perform other diagnostic tests, such as neuroimaging, before genetic tests. These preparatory steps change the differential diagnosis and generate hypotheses that can be tested with more targeted tests.

Phenotype Characterization

Clinicians should try to obtain a clear history of the type, onset, and progression of symptoms in each patient. For NDDs, the trajectory of the neurodevelopmental symptoms (delay, plateau, or regression) may be difficult to elicit when the parental memory of milestones is unreliable or unavailable (eg, foster placement). A review of documented assessments of development and neuropsychological performance in the medical record may be a more objective source of data. Neurologists may need encouragement to review organ systems outside of their area of expertise. A child's medical history may provide clues to multisystem genetic disorders that also affect the brain. A history of recurrent sinus infections in a child with NDD, for example, may lead a clinician to consider a diagnosis of DiGeorge syndrome and its associated thymic hypoplasia and immunodeficiency.[39]

The American Academy of Neurology's practice guideline on the evaluation of children with GDD recommended neuroimaging as part of the workup, with MRI preferred to computed tomography. Such testing is likely to yield abnormal results and to contribute to a diagnosis, even though most of the abnormalities found are nonspecific (atrophy, white matter changes, etc.).[11] Some radiological findings are pathognomonic, such as the pattern of leukoencephalopathy with brain calcifications and cysts that is associated with biallelic variants in SNORD118.[40] Neuroimaging may also be helpful when it is unexpectedly normal, as when it casts additional doubt on a diagnosis of cerebral palsy in a child without a history of significant perinatal distress.[41]

A careful physical examination for minor dysmorphic features can be particularly helpful in generating a hypothesis for a specific genetic syndrome, but many nongeneticists believe that they lack the skill to recognize and describe dysmorphism. Taking a photograph of your patient is often a way to record features that are too difficult to describe. This allows for review at a later date and for collaboration with genetic providers. Experienced geneticists may not be readily available, but computer-assisted facial analysis is available online.[42] One widely used app is Face-2-Gene, which uses an HIPAA-compliant platform to allow health care professionals to aggregate phenotypic information and get suggestions about rare diseases. It can be downloaded at no charge at https://www.face2gene.com/.

A 3-generation pedigree that documents family relationships also reveals patterns of inheritance when other members of the child's family have similar or related features. The University of Iowa offers a helpful tutorial on drawing a pedigree: https://medicine.uiowa.edu/humangenetics/resources/how-draw-pedigree. Parents and grandparents should be asked about their ethnic, geographic, religious (eg, Ashkenazi Jewish), and regional origins as autosomal recessive disorders are more commonly seen in children whose parents share a genetic background.[43] Genetic anticipation, which acts over several generations, provides a clue to the diagnosis of trinucleotide repeat disorders such as fragile X and Huntington disease. This effect is discernible, as symptoms change and become increasingly severe with each generation: for example, in myotonic dystrophy the pedigree can reveal early cataracts in a grandparent, learning disabilities in a mother, and congenital contractures in a newborn.

Choice of Test

Ideally, genetic testing decisions are made after a thorough review of the case history and a careful discussion with the family about the risks, benefits, and limitations of each appropriate testing option. These data can be refined to produce a differential diagnosis (ddx). If the patient exhibits one or more rare features, using them to build a ddx can be an effective strategy. The database of single gene disorders, Online Mendelian Inheritance in Man (https://www.ncbi.nlm.nih.gov/omim), can function as search engine for genetic disorders that match patient features. Using the nonspecific search term "intellectual disability" by itself, returns 1532 results, but when a rare feature such as "molar tooth sign" is added, the list is narrowed to 16 results. If the differential diagnosis is very narrow based on a highly specific phenotype, the genetic test can be similarly focused on one or a few genes.

Single gene and small gene panel tests have advantages. Because they are highly sensitive and specific, with fewer false positives and false negatives, there are fewer ambiguous results to contend with. However, this approach may only be appropriate when the child's phenotype matches a particular syndrome that has a low degree of genetic heterogeneity. For children with nonsyndromic NDDs, both CMA and WES testing are better options with higher yields for pathologic CNVs and SNVs, establishing an etiologic diagnosis 30% to 40% of the time. These genome-wide tests are also more likely to produce false negatives, variants of uncertain significance, and incidental or unrequested abnormalities.

Choosing a genetic test can be complicated when different laboratories offer test menus that are changing constantly. A helpful resource is maintained by the National Center for Biotechnology Information: https://www.ncbi.nlm.nih.gov/gtr/.

Resource Constraints

The increased pressure to maximize efficiency in the clinic and the protocol-driven nature of the electronic medical record have the combined effect of reducing the time spent on an individual patient. For something as complex as a neurodevelopmental disorder, this limits the quality and effectiveness of the diagnostic evaluation. The evaluation that we suggest cannot be accomplished in a 40-minute time slot, so critical pieces of information are lost because the medical system squeezes them out. A thoughtfully designed system can capture some of this information, such as family history, using carefully constructed questionnaires. Breaking the evaluation up into several visits allows for a more comprehensive approach and collaboration with outside experts. Another limiting factor in the United States is the gate-keeping role played by private medical insurance companies that deny authorizations of payment for expensive genetic tests even when they are cost-effective in the long run. As the cost of genetic testing comes down, there will be less justification for this strategy.

INTERPRETATION

Variants of any type are only significant when they occur in disease-causing genes that are relevant to the patient's clinical phenotype. Results need to be interpreted with this in mind. Once identified, SNVs and CNVs are relevant only when they can be associated with disease. Five categories are used to describe variants: pathogenic, likely pathogenic, uncertain, likely benign, and benign.[44] Benign polymorphisms and pathologic mutations are the most easily interpreted variant type because they are unambiguous. Variants are classified as likely benign or likely pathogenic when there is a 90% or greater certainty that the variant is either benign or pathogenic.[44] Follow-up on nearly 600 thousand variants reported to a disease database over a 3-year period found that those listed as "likely pathogenic" were the most likely to be reclassified, with most reclassified as pathogenic, including 70% of those predicted to cause a missense mutation and 90% of those predicted to cause a loss-of-function mutation.[45] Inheritance of a variant from an unaffected parent supports a benign or likely benign categorization.

Genomic tests such as CMA and WES scour the genome for variants and find them at a rate that exceeds our ability to analyze their significance.[46] Clinicians should expect to receive reports with multiple VUS that will need to be carefully reviewed and considered for significance.[47] VUS interpretation takes several factors into account:

- The population frequency of the variant
- The predicted functional effect of the variant on gene expression and protein assembly
- Statistical evidence of the degree to which a nucleotide is conserved in evolution
- The match between the patient and the expected inheritance pattern and phenotype for the gene

Even when a gene is known to be associated with a subject's symptoms, there may be inadequate evidence to classify a VUS as pathogenic. A *de novo* missense mutation may not disrupt the function of a gene whose pathogenicity has previously only been reported with deletion or truncation.[48]

CNVs that are found within regions of the genome without known or well-studied genes are often reported as likely benign, awaiting new information that can assist with reclassification. When a VUS is found, parental testing is recommended to determine whether the variant was inherited or *de novo* in the index subject. Although this testing is certainly instructive, it is not always determinative. Some CNVs are known to have variable expressivity, highly variable phenotypic features, and/or incomplete penetrance, complicating the interpretation of the significance of the CNV for the patient and family.[49]

Variants classified as either pathogenic or likely pathogenic are not found in healthy individuals and thus typically occur as *de novo* mutations. A CNV is more likely to be pathogenic if it contains genes associated with the same clinical phenotype demonstrated by the test subject. A CNV with a high frequency in the population is likely to be a benign polymorphism, but a CNV that has a low frequency or is absent in the population may not be pathogenic.[46] A laboratory may contact the ordering physician if a VUS is reinterpreted as new information comes to light and the responsibility falls to that physician to get in touch with the family or with the current physician caring for the patient. Clinicians should consider requesting reinterpretation of variants of uncertain significance every year or two as new data become available.

Management of VUS should include careful counseling of families with an understanding of the many ways in which the information can be misinterpreted. Plans should be discussed for considering additional or repeat testing to clarify the classification of the variant. A useful resource that curates patient information booklets on common CNVs is https://www.rarechromo.org/. Gene Reviews offers up-to-date evidence-based summaries of many genetic disorders: https://www.ncbi.nlm.nih.gov/books/NBK1116/.

DATABASES

Several well-curated genomic databases organize the ever-growing number of newly discovered DNA variants and their clinical associations. A robust network of easily updated and searchable population, disease-specific, and sequence databases makes it easier for laboratories and clinicians to interpret, classify, and reclassify variants.[50] Population databases facilitate the interpretation of a VUS in light of the frequency with which it occurs in large populations. Two large-scale population databases currently in widespread use by laboratories are the ExAC and gnomAD projects.[51,52] Researchers and clinicians can securely submit patient information to these and other disease databases, including ClinVar, dGV, and dbVar.[53–55]

Disease databases make it easier to gauge the likely pathogenicity of variants found in patients with a similar phenotype. One disease-related database, Database of Chromosomal Imbalance and Phenotype in Humans using Ensembl Resources, includes the Developmental Disorder Genotype-Phenotype Database, which is a curated list of more than 2000 genes reported to be associated with NDD, categorized by level of certainty of the association and the allelic status associated with disease (monoallelic, biallelic, etc): https://decipher.sanger.ac.uk/ddd#ddgenes.

ETHICAL CONSIDERATIONS

Many of the ethical considerations associated with genetic testing can be addressed with thorough pretest counseling and informed consenting. The potential pitfalls include the following:

- Interpretation of a positive result as a reason for feeling guilt or placing blame
- Loss of patient privacy when identifying clinical information is posted to a public database
- Identification of abnormal results in family members tested to classify a variant of uncertain significance
- Parental misidentification (adoption, gamete donation) and unexpected consanguinity/incest

Patients and their families are prone to misinterpret the results of a genetic test, even when appropriate counseling has been provided. Nonphysicians are more likely to view genetics as rigidly deterministic and to have less familiarity with concepts of scientific uncertainty. Patients, their families, and occasionally their health care providers may be so invested in having a positive test end a long and difficult "diagnostic odyssey" that they consider a VUS to be pathologic despite counseling to the contrary.[49] Parents who receive a negative genetic test result may even feel an unexpected sense of relief, realizing, in retrospect, that a genetic explanation would have made them feel responsible for their child's symptoms and would have denied them hope for a cause more amenable to treatment.[49]

Informed consent should precede genetic testing for neurodevelopmental disorders.[56] Proper informed consent should review the implications of test results and how the family will perceive them, whether positive, negative, or inconclusive. The family should feel that they have an adequate understanding of the risks and benefits before deciding the degree to which they want unsolicited information about pathologic variants shared with them. Positive genetic test results can result in changes in therapy service eligibility, insurance discrimination, and increased fear and stigmatization. Adolescents with the capacity to participate in the decision-making process should also consent to genetic testing. Their feelings and opinions about testing should be sought out and respected.[57,58]

Even a microarray can reveal sensitive information. Long stretches of homozygosity, in the context of a young mother, especially one who is a minor herself, implicates not only incest but sexual abuse by a male relative and should prompt a broader investigation by police, social services, or child protection agencies. With this sobering thought in mind, the clinician should always counsel the family before testing in order to anticipate problems that may arise, including the following:

- The results can be normal, may show a clearly benign or clearly pathogenic CNV, or may show a variant of uncertain or uncertain significance, as is reported in up to 20% of studies. VUS are even more likely in patients of non-European descent, due to a still extant latency in compiling variant databases in non-European populations.[47]
- The results may reveal a CNV that predisposes to adult-onset conditions for which there may or may not be available treatments
- Testing may reveal unexpected nonpaternity/nonmaternity or consanguinity
- Family members may need to be tested to fully determine the significance of findings, and the results may have implications for their own health or reproductive risks
- Testing will not affect health insurance eligibility but may have an effect on applications for other forms of insurance
- Interpretation of test results may change in the future as new information is obtained
- Repeat testing with the same or alternative methods may be needed to clarify results
- A referral to a Genetics clinic may be needed for counseling or test interpretation
- Some genetic abnormalities cannot be identified by CMA. Mosaicism, balanced translocations, sequence variants, mitochondrial DNA variants, and trinucleotide repeat disorders such as fragile X syndrome are only likely to be detected with targeted testing.

FUTURE DIRECTIONS

It can be anticipated that WES and WGS will eventually supplant the use of CMA techniques.[59] Ongoing refinements of NGS techniques are already substantially improving coverage of functional domains, sensitivity for copy number changes and copy-neutral rearrangements, and resolution of areas with repetitive sequences. Advances in information processing and automated variant calling, filtering, and classification will lead to further reductions in the price of genome-wide testing, including WGS, making NGS tests available for an even larger pool of patients for whom testing remains out of reach for financial considerations. Further research is expected to confirm current recommendations that NGS testing replaces other genetic tests as the first-line tool for evaluating neurodevelopmental disorders of unknown cause.[23] Additional studies are likely to show higher yields as test characteristics and databases improve, with greater impact on clinical management as more gene-specific treatments are developed. Further cost-analysis research is likely to show that NGS, when it replaces an extensive battery of expensive and invasive tests, proves to be cost-effective as a first-line diagnostic test for many neurologic disorders, including developmental disabilities.[60,61]

Many of the clinicians who routinely evaluate children presenting with neurodevelopmental disorders and CA have little formal training in genetics, particularly in pretest counseling and in the interpretation and investigation of VUS. It is unlikely that a sufficient quantity of medical geneticists and counselors will ever be available to fully meet the increasing demands for their expertise, even with creative restructuring to provide services on a regional basis.[62] The situation frequently results in the underutilization, misapplication, and misinterpretation of available tests and in the dissatisfaction and frustration of patients and their families.[63,64] Research is focusing on developing better approaches to educational materials and best practices for relaying genetic information to families.[65] The BYOG strategy (Become Your Own Geneticist) may be the practical solution by incorporating and integrating genetics education into the lifelong training of generalists and specialists of all types.

Continued coordination between clinicians, researchers, and large genetics laboratories around the world will increase participation of non-European subjects in population databases and improve the interpretation of results in all racial and ethnic groups. Data integration will become increasingly challenging as NGS becomes more accessible, and data of increasing complexity are collected. Millions of new variants from coding and noncoding regions will be correlated with detailed patient and family histories. Variants will be more easily classified, with fewer uncertainties. New causal associations for specific diseases, with both Mendelian and polygenetic inheritance patterns, will be incorporated into our knowledge base. Interfaces designed to search and analyze these pooled data will become more user-friendly.[66]

The possibilities for personalized treatment afforded by genetic diagnosis are actively driving research and promise to revolutionize clinical medicine. As our understanding of allele-specific pathogenicity is further refined to include gain-of-function or loss-of-function effects, treatment strategies will be tailored not just to a particular diagnosis but to a particular allele. In an illustrative example, Dravet syndrome, when caused by a toxic gain-of-function variant in one *SCN1A* allele, has been treated effectively with an antisense oligonucleotide in a mouse model.[67] There will be more of this to come.

SUMMARY

Remarkable progress has occurred within clinical genetics in the 20 years since the publication of the first human genome. As genetic testing methods have become more cost-effective and powerful, genetic tests have become more informative and more widely used, even as major challenges remain in test implementation and interpretation. Modern genetic tests are increasingly likely to provide a diagnosis for patients with unexplained NDDs and CA, yielding numerous benefits for them and their families. However, these tests also have an increased likelihood of generating results that are of uncertain significance and that require judicious analysis, additional testing, and long-term follow-up. Efforts to improve and standardize data processing and case resolution are ongoing within the research and genetics community. There is an as yet unmet need for genetic training for clinicians at every level, as genetics plays an increasingly prominent role in appropriate test application and interpretation in medicine.

REFERENCES

1. Sherr EH, Michelson DJ, Shevell MI, et al. Neurodevelopment disorders and genetic testing: current approaches and future advances. Ann Neurol 2013;72: 164–70. Available at: https://onlinelibrary.wiley.com/doi/full/10.1002/ana.23950.

2. American Psychiatric Association. Diagnostic and statistical manual of mental disorders: diagnostic and statistical manual of mental disorders. 5th edition. Arlington (VA): American Psychiatric Association; 2013.

3. Boat TF, Wu JT. Clinical characteristics of intellectual disabilities. Mental disorders and disabilities among low-income children. Washington, DC: The National Academic Press; 2015.

4. Sharma SR, Gonda X, Tarazi FI. Autism spectrum disorder: classification, diagnosis and therapy. Pharmacol Ther 2018;190:91–104. Available at: https://www.sciencedirect.com/science/article/pii/S0163725818300871?via%3Dihub.

5. Volkmar FR, McPartland JC. From Kanner to DSM-5: autism as an evolving diagnostic concept. Annu Rev Clin Psychol 2014;10:193–212. Available at: https://www.annualreviews.org/doi/10.1146/annurev-clinpsy-032813-153710.

6. Lukmanji S, Manji SA, Kadhim S, et al. The co-occurrence of epilepsy and autism: a systematic review. Epilepsy Behav 2019;98(Pt A):238–48. Available at: https://www.sciencedirect.com/science/article/pii/S1525505019304949?via%3Dihub.

7. CDC website. Available at: https://www.cdc.gov/ncbddd/birthdefects/surveillancemanual/appendices/appendix-c.html. Accessed November 23, 2019.

8. D'Arrigo S, Gavazzi F, Alfei E, et al. The diagnostic yield of array comparative genomic hybridization is high regardless of severity of intellectual disability/developmental delay in children. J Child Neurol 2016;31:691–9. Available at: https://journals.sagepub.com/doi/10.1177/0883073815613562.

9. Miller DT, Adam MP, Aradhya S, et al. Consensus statement: chromosomal microarray is a first-tier clinical diagnostic test for individuals with developmental disabilities or congenital anomalies. Am J Hum Genet 2010;86(5):749–64. Available at: https://www.sciencedirect.com/science/article/pii/S0002929710002089?via%3Dihub.

10. Flore LA, Milunsky JM. Updates in the genetic evaluation of the child with global developmental delay or intellectual disability. Semin Pediatr Neurol 2012;19: 173–80. Available at: https://www.sciencedirect.com/science/article/pii/S1071909112000721?via%3Dihub.

11. Shevell M, Ashwal S, Donley D, et al. Practice parameter: evaluation of the child with global developmental delay: report of the quality standards subcommittee of the American Academy of Neurology and The Practice Committee of the Child Neurology Society. Neurology 2003;60:367–80. Available at: https://n.neurology.org/content/60/3/367.

12. Hochstenbach R, Slunga-Tallberg A, Devlin C, et al. Fading competency of cytogenetic diagnostic laboratories: the alarm bell has started to ring. Eur J Hum Genet 2017;25(3):273–4. Available at: https://www.nature.com/articles/ejhg2016177.

13. Beaudet AL. The utility of chromosomal microarray analysis in developmental and behavioral pediatrics. Child Dev 2013;84:121–32. Available at: https://www.ncbi.nlm.nih.gov/pmc/articles/PMC3725967/.

14. Boone PM, Bacino CA, Shaw CA, et al. Detection of clinically relevant exonic copy-number changes by array CGH. Hum Mutat 2010;31:1326–42. Available at: https://www.ncbi.nlm.nih.gov/pmc/articles/PMC3158569/.

15. Schaaf CP, Wiszniewska J, Beaudet AL. Copy number and SNP arrays in clinical diagnostics. Annu Rev Genomics Hum Genet 2011;12:25–51. Available at: https://www.annualreviews.org/doi/10.1146/annurev-genom-092010-110715.

16. Tan WH, Bird LM, Thibert RL, et al. If not Angelman, what is it? A review of Angelman-like syndromes. Am J Med Genet A 2014;164A(4):975–92. Available at: https://onlinelibrary.wiley.com/doi/full/10.1002/ajmg.a.36416.

17. Hayward BE, Kumari D, Usdin K. Recent advances in assays for the fragile X-related disorders. Hum Genet 2017;136(10):1313–27. Available at: https://www.ncbi.nlm.nih.gov/pmc/articles/PMC5769695/.

18. Aref-Eshghi E, Bend EG, Colaiacovo S, et al. Diagnostic utility of genome-wide DNA methylation testing in genetically unsolved individuals with suspected hereditary conditions. Am J Hum Genet 2019;104(4):685–700. Available at: https://www.ncbi.nlm.nih.gov/pmc/articles/PMC6451739/.

19. Barros-Silva D, Marques CJ, Henrique R, et al. Profiling DNA methylation based on next-generation sequencing approaches: new insights and clinical applications. Genes (Basel) 2018;9(9) [pii:E429]. Available at: https://www.ncbi.nlm.nih.gov/pmc/articles/PMC6162482/.

20. Aspromonte MC, Bellini M, Gasparini A, et al. Characterization of intellectual disability and autism comorbidity through gene panel sequencing. Hum Mutat 2019;40(9):1346–63. Available at: https://onlinelibrary.wiley.com/doi/full/10.1002/humu.23822.

21. Venter JC, Adams MD, Myers EW, et al. The sequence of the human genome. Science 2001;291(5507):1304–51. Available at: https://science.sciencemag.org/content/291/5507/1304.

22. Warr A, Robert C, Hume D, et al. Exome sequencing: current and future perspectives. G3 (Bethesda) 2015;5:1543–50. Available at: https://www.ncbi.nlm.nih.gov/pmc/articles/PMC4528311/.

23. Srivastava S, Love-Nichols JA, Dies KA, et al. Meta-analysis and multidisciplinary consensus statement: exome sequencing is a first-tier clinical diagnostic test for individuals with neurodevelopmental disorders. Genet Med 2019;21(11):2413–21. Available at: https://www.ncbi.nlm.nih.gov/pmc/articles/PMC6831729/.

24. Behjati S, Tarpey PS. What is next generation sequencing? Arch Dis Child 2013;98:236–8. Available at: https://www.ncbi.nlm.nih.gov/pmc/articles/PMC3841808/.

25. Baldridge D, Heeley J, Vineyard M, et al. The Exome Clinic and the role of medical genetics expertise in the interpretation of exome sequencing results. Genet Med 2017;19(9):1040–8. Available at: https://www.ncbi.nlm.nih.gov/pmc/articles/PMC5581723/.

26. Shigemizu D, Momozawa Y, Abe T, et al. Performance comparison of four commercial human whole-exome capture platforms. Sci Rep 2015;5:12742. Available at: https://www.ncbi.nlm.nih.gov/pmc/articles/PMC4522667/.

27. Whitford W, Lehnert K, Snell RG, et al. Evaluation of the performance of copy number variant prediction tools for the detection of deletions from whole genome sequencing data. J Biomed Inform 2019;94:103174. Available at: https://www.sciencedirect.com/science/article/pii/S1532046419300929?via%3Dihub.

28. Landry LG, Ali N, Williams DR, et al. Lack of diversity in genomic databases is a barrier to translating precision medicine research into practice. Health Aff (Millwood) 2018;37(5):780–5. Available at: https://www.healthaffairs.org/doi/10.1377/hlthaff.2017.1595.

29. Clark MM, Stark Z, Farnaes L, et al. Meta-analysis of the diagnostic and clinical utility of genome and exome sequencing and chromosomal microarray in children with suspected genetic diseases. NPJ Genom Med 2018;3:16. Available at: https://www.ncbi.nlm.nih.gov/pmc/articles/PMC6037748/.

30. Mu XJ, Lu ZJ, Kong Y, et al. Analysis of genomic variation in non-coding elements using population-scale sequencing data from the 1000 Genomes Project. Nucleic

Acids Res 2011;39(16):7058–76. Available at: https://www.ncbi.nlm.nih.gov/pmc/articles/PMC3167619/.

31. Ward LD, Kellis M. Interpreting noncoding genetic variation in complex traits and human disease. Nat Biotechnol 2012;30(11):1095–106. Available at: https://www.ncbi.nlm.nih.gov/pmc/articles/PMC3703467/.

32. Botstein D, Risch N. Discovering genotypes underlying human phenotypes: past successes for mendelian disease, future approaches for complex disease. Nat Genet 2003;33(Suppl):228–37. Available at: https://www.nature.com/articles/ng1090z.

33. Khurana E, Fu Y, Colonna V, et al. Integrative annotation of variants from 1092 humans: application to cancer genomics. Science 2013;342(6154):1235587. Available at: https://www.ncbi.nlm.nih.gov/pmc/articles/PMC3947637/.

34. Schluth-Bolard C, Diguet F, Chatron N, et al. Whole genome paired-end sequencing elucidates functional and phenotypic consequences of balanced chromosomal rearrangement in patients with developmental disorders. J Med Genet 2019;56(8):526–35. Available at: https://jmg.bmj.com/content/56/8/526.

35. Dong Z, Ye L, Yang Z, et al. Balanced chromosomal rearrangement detection by low-pass whole-genome sequencing. Curr Protoc Hum Genet 2018;96: 8.18.1–8.18.16. Available at: https://www.ncbi.nlm.nih.gov/pmc/articles/PMC5924704/.

36. Parikh S, Goldstein A, Koenig MK, et al. Diagnosis and management of mitochondrial disease: a consensus statement from the Mitochondrial Medicine Society. Genet Med 2015;17(9):689–701. Available at: https://www.ncbi.nlm.nih.gov/pmc/articles/PMC5000852/.

37. Duan M, Chen L, Ge Q, et al. Evaluating heteroplasmic variations of the mitochondrial genome from whole genome sequencing data. Gene 2019;699: 145–54. Available at: https://www.sciencedirect.com/science/article/pii/S0378111919302422?via%3Dihub.

38. van Dijk EL, Jaszczyszyn Y, Naquin D, et al. The third revolution in sequencing technology. Trends Genet 2018;34(9):666–81. Available at: https://www.sciencedirect.com/science/article/pii/S0168952518300969?via%3Dihub.

39. Morsheimer M, Brown Whitehorn TF, Heimall J, et al. The immune deficiency of chromosome 22q11.2 deletion syndrome. Am J Med Genet A 2017;173(9): 2366–72. Available at: https://onlinelibrary.wiley.com/doi/full/10.1002/ajmg.a.38319.

40. Hermens M, van der Knaap MS, Kamsteeg EJ, et al. A brother and sister with intellectual disability and characteristic neuroimaging findings. Eur J Paediatr Neurol 2018;22(5):866–9. Available at: https://www.sciencedirect.com/science/article/pii/S1090379818302095?via%3Dihub.

41. Pearson TS, Pons R, Ghaoui R, et al. Genetic mimics of cerebral palsy. Mov Disord 2019;34(5):625–36. Available at: https://onlinelibrary.wiley.com/doi/full/10.1002/mds.27655.

42. Zarate YA, Bosanko KA, Gripp KW. Using facial analysis technology in a typical genetic clinic: experience from 30 individuals from a single institution. J Hum Genet 2019;64(12):1243–5. Available at: https://www.nature.com/articles/s10038-019-0673-6.

43. Çaksen H, Aktar F, Yıldırım G, et al. Importance of pedigree in patients with familial epilepsy and intellectual disability. Sudan J Paediatr 2019;19(1):52–6. Available at: https://www.ncbi.nlm.nih.gov/pmc/articles/PMC6589802/.

44. Richards S, Aziz N, Bale S, et al. Standards and guidelines for the interpretation of sequence variants: a joint consensus recommendation of the American

College of Medical Genetics and Genomics and the Association for Molecular Pathology. Genet Med 2015;17:405–24. Available at: https://www.ncbi.nlm.nih.gov/pmc/articles/PMC4544753/.

45. Harrison SM, Rehm HL. Is 'likely pathogenic' really 90% likely? Reclassification data in ClinVar. Genome Med 2019;11(1):72. Available at: https://genomemedicine.biomedcentral.com/articles/10.1186/s13073-019-0688-9.

46. Duzkale H, Shen J, McLaughlin H, et al. A systemicatic approach to assessing the clinical significance of genetic variants. Clin Genet 2013;84:453–63. Available at: https://www.ncbi.nlm.nih.gov/pmc/articles/PMC3995020/.

47. Hoffman-Andrews L. The known unknown: the challenges of genetic variants of uncertain significance in clinical practice. J Law Biosci 2017;4:648–57. Available at: https://www.ncbi.nlm.nih.gov/pmc/articles/PMC5965500/.

48. Vears DF, Sénécal K, Borry P. Reporting practices for variants of uncertain significance from next generation sequencing technologies. Eur J Med Genet 2017; 60(10):553–8. Available at: https://www.sciencedirect.com/science/article/pii/S1769721217302653?via%3Dihub.

49. Reiff M, Bernhardt BA, Mulchandani S, et al. What does it mean?": uncertainties in understanding results of chromosomal microarray testing. Genet Med 2012; 14(2):250–8. Available at: https://www.ncbi.nlm.nih.gov/pmc/articles/PMC3445036/.

50. Katsanis SH, Katsanis N. Molecular genetic testing and the future of clinical genomics. Nat Rev Genet 2013,14(6):415 26. Available at: https://www.ncbi.nlm.nih.gov/pmc/articles/PMC4461364/.

51. Lek M, Karczewski KJ, Minikel EV, et al. Analysis of protein-coding genetic variation in 60,706 humans. Nature 2016;536:285–91. Available at: https://www.ncbi.nlm.nih.gov/pmc/articles/PMC5018207/.

52. Karczewski KJ, Francioli LC, Tiao G. The mutational constraint spectrum quantified from variation in 141,456 humans. Nature 2020;581: 434-3. Available at: https://doi.org/10.1038/s41586-020-2308-7.

53. Landrum MJ, Lee JM, Benson M, et al. ClinVar: improving access to variant interpretation and supporting evidence. Nucleic Acids Res 2018;46:D1062–7. Available at: https://www.ncbi.nlm.nih.gov/pmc/articles/PMC5753237/.

54. MacDonald JR, Ziman R, Yuen RK, et al. The Database of Genomic Variants: a curated collection of structural variation in the human genome. Nucleic Acids Res 2014;42(Database issue):D986–92. Available at: https://www.ncbi.nlm.nih.gov/pmc/articles/PMC3965079/.

55. Lappalainen I, Lopez J, Skipper L, et al. DbVar and DGVa: public archives for genomic structural variation. Nucleic Acids Res 2013;41:936–41. Available at: https://www.ncbi.nlm.nih.gov/pmc/articles/PMC3531204/.

56. McKay V, Efron D, Palmer EE, et al. Current use of chromosomal microarray by Australian paediatricians and implications for the implementation of next generation sequencing. J Paediatr Child Health 2017;53(7):650–6. Available at: https://onlinelibrary.wiley.com/doi/full/10.1111/jpc.13523.

57. Ross LF, Saal HM, David KL, et al. Technical report: ethical and policy issues in genetic testing and screening of children. Genet Med 2013;15:234–45. Available at: https://www.nature.com/articles/gim2012176.

58. Bush LW, Bartoshesky LE, David KL, et al. Pediatric clinical exome/genome sequencing and the engagement process: encouraging active conversation with the older child and adolescent: points to consider - a statement of the American College of Medical Genetics and Genomics (ACMG). Genet Med 2018;20: 692–4. Available at: https://www.nature.com/articles/gim201836.

59. Rosenfeld JA, Patel A. Chromosomal microarrays: understanding genetics of neurodevelopmental disorders and congenital anomalies. J Pediatr Genet 2017;6(1):42–50. Available at: https://www.ncbi.nlm.nih.gov/pmc/articles/PMC5288005/.

60. Marques Matos C, Alonso I, Leão M. Diagnostic yield of next-generation sequencing applied to neurological disorders. J Clin Neurosci 2019;67:14–8. Available at: https://www.sciencedirect.com/science/article/pii/S0967586818321258?via%3Dihub.

61. Nolan D, Carlson M. Whole exome sequencing in pediatric neurology patients: clinical implications and estimated cost analysis. J Child Neurol 2016; 31(7):887–94. Available at: https://journals.sagepub.com/doi/10.1177/0883073815627880.

62. Kaye C, Bodurtha J, Edick M, et al. Regional models of genetic services in the United States. Genet Med 2019;22(2):381–8. Available at: https://www.nature.com/articles/s41436-019-0648-1.

63. Kiely B, Vettam S, Adesman A. Utilization of genetic testing among children with developmental disabilities in the United States. Appl Clin Genet 2016;9:93–100. Available at: https://www.ncbi.nlm.nih.gov/pmc/articles/PMC4946856/.

64. Zhao S, Chen WJ, Dhar SU, et al. Genetic testing experiences among parents of children with autism spectrum disorder in the United States. J Autism Dev Disord 2019;49(12):4821–33. Available at: https://link.springer.com/article/10.1007%2Fs10803-019-04200-z.

65. Jez S, Martin M, South S, et al. Variants of unknown significance on chromosomal microarray analysis: parental perspectives. J Community Genet 2015;6(4):343–9. Available at: https://www.ncbi.nlm.nih.gov/pmc/articles/PMC4567987/.

66. Nellåker C, Alkuraya FS, Baynam G, et al. Minerva consortium. enabling global clinical collaborations on identifiable patient data: the minerva initiative. Front Genet 2019;10:611. Available at: https://www.ncbi.nlm.nih.gov/pmc/articles/PMC6681681/.

67. Perry MS. New and emerging medications for treatment of pediatric epilepsy. Pediatr Neurol 2019. https://doi.org/10.1016/j.pediatrneurol.2019.11.008 [pii:S0887-8994(19)30923-3]. Available at: https://www.ncbi.nlm.nih.gov/pubmed/31980296.

Proteopathic Seed Amplification Assays for Neurodegenerative Disorders

Natália do Carmo Ferreira, PhD, Byron Caughey, PhD*

KEYWORDS

• Seed • PMCA • RT-QuIC • Prion • Synuclein • Tau • β-Amyloid • Biomarkers

KEY POINTS

- Prion-like, self-propagating protein aggregates can cause, and serve as biomarkers for, multiple neurodegenerative diseases.
- The seeded polymerization growth mechanism of pathologic protein aggregates has been exploited to develop ultrasensitive assays for many of these biomarkers.
- Some of these types of assays (eg, prion and α-synuclein real-time quaking-induced conversion assays), can provide highly sensitive and specific diagnoses of prion diseases and α-synucleinopathies when applied to patients' cerebrospinal fluid or nasal brushings.
- Multiple ultrasensitive seed amplification assays have also been developed for many disease-associated types of tau and Aβ aggregates in biospecimens, but these assays are in earlier stages of diagnostic evaluation.
- The development of a broad panel of proteopathic seed amplification biomarker assays should facilitate the diagnosis of neurodegenerative diseases as well as the execution of clinical trials of potential therapeutics.

INTRODUCTION

In order to function properly, proteins typically must fold and assume defined native three-dimensional structures. However, disruption of native protein folding may allow abnormal aggregation into self-propagating assemblies (seeds) that can grow by recruiting, and misfolding, additional monomers. Such protein aggregates can be more toxic[1,2] or more infectious[3] when small (oligomeric), but continued growth can result in the accumulation of highly ordered amyloid fibrils, and bundles thereof, that comprise the pathologic protein deposits that often characterize protein misfolding diseases.[4] Protein quality control (proteostasis) mechanisms usually limit the accumulation of abnormally folded and aggregated proteins.[5] However, with aging,

Laboratory of Persistent Viral Diseases, Rocky Mountain Laboratories, National Institute for Allergy and Infectious Diseases, National Institutes of Health, 903 South 4th Street, Hamilton, MT 59840, USA
* Corresponding author.
E-mail address: bcaughey@nih.gov

Clin Lab Med 40 (2020) 257–270
https://doi.org/10.1016/j.cll.2020.04.002
0272-2712/20/Published by Elsevier Inc.

pathogenic mutations in specific proteins, inoculation of preformed seeds, or perhaps other factors, protein quality control mechanisms can be overwhelmed, allowing protein aggregation to spiral out of control. The accumulation of protein aggregates may, or may not, have devastating consequences for the host.[6]

Nervous tissue, with its lack of neuronal turnover, is particularly vulnerable to the effects of pathologic protein aggregation. The aggregation of specific proteins is known to feature prominently in the pathogenesis of many neurodegenerative diseases, including Alzheimer disease (AD), Parkinson disease (PD), and prion diseases.[1] In genetic forms of these diseases, mutated proteins seem to be more prone to aggregation, leading to the appearance of neurodegenerative disorders in earlier stages of life. Considering the relative inability of neurons to regenerate, accurate diagnosis in the early stages of these diseases should facilitate effective treatment while neuronal damage is not yet too extensive and/or irreversible. In this context, proteopathic seed amplification assays have provided means of detecting minute amounts (attograms to femtograms) of self-propagating protein aggregates in diverse biological specimens by exploiting their inherent seeded polymerization growth mechanisms.[7–15]

The assembly of proteins into amyloid fibrils is akin to one-dimensional crystallization.[16] As with other crystallizations, the de novo, or spontaneous, formation of seeds in a solution of monomers usually takes much longer than the growth of preexisting seeds. In proteopathic seed amplification assays, a biospecimen is incubated in the presence of a vast stoichiometric excess of soluble protein monomers under appropriate conditions. If the specimen contains seeds, the assembly of monomers into amyloid fibrils occurs more rapidly than the de novo assembly that eventually occurs in the absence of seeds. Thus, seeds can be detected by comparing lag phases, or the reaction times required to detect amyloid that is newly formed from the monomeric substrate molecules. This use of substrate is analogous to the substrate in an enzymatic reaction rather than to a structure onto which something builds. Because the substrate molecules are much more abundant than the seeds in a biospecimen, their conversion into amyloid fibrils can, in effect, provide billion-fold, or even trillion-fold amplifications of the seed.[17,18] Such amplification can enable ultrasensitive detection of even a few seed particles in a test sample. This article highlights many of these types of assays, with an emphasis on their applications to human proteopathies.

PRION SEED AMPLIFICATION ASSAYS

The most highly developed proteopathic seed amplification assays are those for prions, with current assays allowing highly accurate molecular diagnoses of prion diseases in living patients.[15,19–21] The ability of infectious prions to induce the conversion of natively folded prion protein (PrP^C) into a prion-like protease-resistant form (PrP^{res}) in a cell-free system was first demonstrated in 1994.[22] This experimental system revealed prion strain and sequence specificities of this prion-seeded conversion reaction,[23–27] but did not support the continuous prion propagation that would be required for an amplification assay.

Protein Misfolding Cyclic Amplification

Several years later Soto and coworkers[7] developed a highly sensitive PrP^{Sc} (infectious scrapie prion protein [PrP]) amplification method termed protein misfolding cyclic amplification (PMCA).[7] In this assay, attogram amounts of PrP^{Sc} present in a tissue sample can be amplified to detectable levels by its incubation with an excess of noninfected brain homogenate, which provides the PrP^C monomers needed for the polymerization process. By interleaving incubation and sonication steps, the newly synthesized misfolded aggregate is intermittently broken, providing more seeds, amplifying PrP^{res} and prion infectivity exponentially. The final product is then subjected to a proteinase K (PK) treatment and proteinase-resistant fragments are revealed by Western blotting with an anti-PrP antibody. PrP^{Sc} can be amplified from a 10^{-12} dilution of infected hamster brain homogenate containing ~26 PrP^{Sc} molecules.[17] A key feature of PMCA is that it faithfully replicates the PrP^{Sc} structure such that the amplified products are fully infectious.[28,29] Thus, PMCA has been invaluable as an in vitro experimental system for studying prion propagation. In contrast, infectious prion amplification can be a disadvantage for routine diagnostic applications when it would be preferable not to generate large amounts of infectivity. Notwithstanding that practical concern, PMCA has clear diagnostic potential because prions have been amplified from blood samples of experimentally infected animals at late[30] and early[31] stages of the disease, as well as in urine samples from animals[32] and humans with variant Creutzfeldt-Jakob disease (CJD).[33]

To circumvent the need to use brain homogenates as a source of PrP^C substrate, Atarashi and colleagues[8] developed PMCA reaction conditions that allowed the use of bacterially expressed recombinant PrP^C as the reaction substrate. This assay was called rPrP PMCA and allowed the detection of attogram-range amounts of PrP^{Sc} in 2 to 3 days compared with the 2 to 3 weeks required for conventional PMCA assays at that time. A subsequent rPrP PMCA permutation called quaking-induced conversion (QuIC) allowed the substitution of more reproducible shaking for sonication.[12]

Amyloid Seeding Assay

Meanwhile, Colby and colleagues[9] also developed a highly sensitive assay for PrP^{Sc} using recombinant PrP^C as a substrate, called the amyloid seeding assay (ASA). The ASA, which was also shaken rather than sonicated, had the major practical advantages of having a multiwell plate–based assay format and a direct fluorescence readout. The basic principle was that PrP^{Sc} seeds in a sample could induce the formation of recombinant PrP amyloid fibrils, which were then detected with the amyloid-sensitive dye thioflavin T (ThT). Frequent fluorescence measurements while the reactions progressed in a shaking fluorescence plate reader allowed convenient measurement of the relative lag phases of reactions seeded with prion-infected (eg, sporadic CJD [sCJD]) versus negative control brain homogenates. However, in contrast with most RT-QuIC assays, a phosphotungstate-precipitation step was needed in order to purify the seeds before its use in the ASA.

Real-Time Quaking-Induced Conversion

By combining various aspects of the QuIC and ASA assays and further optimizations, Atarashi and colleagues[10] developed the first real-time (RT) QuIC assays (**Fig. 1**), which provided easier distinction of prion-infected and uninfected biospecimens such as cerebrospinal fluid (CSF),[10,11] often without the need of doing a preclearing of the sample. Many laboratories have since contributed to the development of assays for most known prions of mammals (eg, Ref.[34–36] and references therein). The analytical sensitivities of these assays often reach down in the low femtogram to attogram range and typically meet or markedly exceed the sensitivities of animal bioassays for prions. RT-QuIC assays have been adapted to diverse tissues and biological fluids, including brain, skin, olfactory mucosa, blood, CSF, saliva, urine, and feces.[18,33,37–45] Faster and more sensitive second-generation RT-QuIC assays for human prions allow nearly 100% accurate antemortem diagnosis of sCJD when CSF, nasal brushings, or both are tested.[21,41,46] Analysis of CSF specimens alone provide 92% to 96% overall

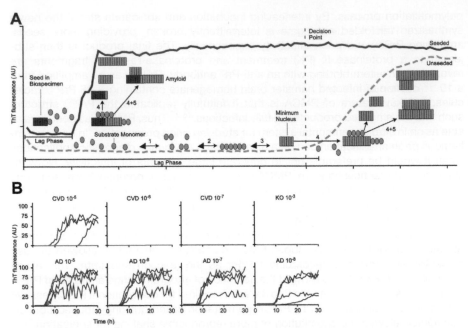

Fig. 1. Seeded polymerization in real-time quaking-induced conversion (RT-QuIC) reactions. (A) Reactions are set up in multiwell plates by diluting a biospecimen into reaction mixture containing a vast stoichiometric excess of an appropriate protein monomer (substrate) for the type of disease-associated seed being detected. The reaction also contains the amyloid-sensitive fluorescent dye, thioflavin T (ThT). When seeds are present in the bio-specimen (*left*), they immediately start to grow (4) by recruiting new monomers. Elongated fibrils can promote secondary nucleation (5); that is, the production of new seeding surfaces either by fragmentation or by providing lateral surfaces that can facilitate the ordering and conformational conversion of monomers into additional fibrils. Secondary nucleation contributes to the exponential growth of the new amyloid that enhances ThT fluorescence (*dark blue trace*). The lag phase in a seeded reaction represents the time it takes for the seeded amyloids to accumulate to levels that are detectable with ThT. Eventually, the reaction plateaus when all of the available monomer is converted to amyloid. In the absence of seeds in a negative control biospecimen (*light blue trace*), spontaneous nucleation (1–3) may occur, but only after a prolonged lag phase during which the kinetically unfavorable process of forming minimal stable nuclei (in this case a 6-mer) occurs.[16] A key to developing an effective assay is finding substrates and assay conditions giving the greatest fold separation between the lag phases of seeded versus unseeded reactions (eg, see Ref.[79]). (B) Representative primary Alzheimer disease (AD) tau RT-QuIC data comparing seeding by serial 10-fold dilutions of human familial AD (age 44 years) and cerebrovascular disease (CVD; age 53 years) brain tissue with reference to a 10^0 dilution being solid brain tissue. Tau knockout (KO) mouse brain served as a completely tau-free negative control. Traces from quadruplicate wells for each brain dilution are shown. AD brain could be diluted at least 10^5-fold and 10^3-fold further than the KO and CVD brains, respectively, and still seed positive reactions. Although the CVD brain was not recorded as having tau pathology by immunohistochemistry, the typically higher sensitivity of RT-QuIC assays likely allowed detection of tau aggregates that were less than the detection limit of immunohistochemistry. AU, arbitrary units.

diagnostic sensitivity (the percentage of patients with sCJD giving positive assays) and nearly 100% specificity (the percentage of patients with nonprion disease giving negative assays) in multiple independent studies by different research groups.[21,40,41,46,47] Before the availability of these assays, definite diagnoses of CJD required biochemical or immunohistologic analysis of brain tissue, which is usually only available postmortem. According to the US Centers for Disease Control and Prevention (CDC), a positive RT-QuIC result in combination with neuropsychiatric symptoms provides a probable diagnosis of CJD, although immunodetection of PrP[res] is still needed for a definite diagnosis.[48] Similar diagnostic criteria are used by the UK National CJD Research and Surveillance Unit.[49] Recent demonstrations of the detection of sCJD prions in the skin[43] and multiple components of the eyes[50] of all tested patients with sCJD have raised the possibility that these tissues might also be useful diagnostically, as well as being potentially biohazardous sources of prion infectivity. Studies in prion-infected rodents have shown that prion seeding activity can be detected in skin far in advance of the onset of overt clinical signs of prion disease.[38] From a practical perspective, concerns have been raised about whether the massively amplified products of sCJD-seeded RT-QuIC assay products are infectious, and therefore biohazardous. However, inoculation of the products of sCJD MM1-seeded RT-QuIC reactions into transgenic mice overexpressing human PrP[C] showed that they were at least 10^{10}-fold less infectious per unit protein than the sCJD prions that seeded its aggregation.[51] Detailed protocols for performing prion RT-QuIC assays have been reported elsewhere.[20,52]

Scrapie Cell Assay

Klohn and colleagues[53] described a prototypic cellular seeding assay that exploits the ability of prions to infect cells and induce the de novo accumulation of PrP[Sc]. Briefly, neuroblastoma-derived cell lines are incubated with dilutions of prion-infected brain homogenates from rodents, and the proportion of cells accumulating PrP[Sc] (detected by an enzyme-linked immune absorbent spot assay after 3 in vitro passages over ~2 weeks total) were found to correlate with the prion concentration in the original sample. The standard scrapie cell assay has been automated[54,55] and is as sensitive as the mouse prion bioassay but is faster and less expensive, with the advantage of no use of animals. There have been many revealing applications of the scrapie cell assay (eg, Refs.[55–57]); however, so far the assay has been limited to the measurement of rodent-adapted prion strains. To date, no scrapie cell assay has been adapted for the detection of human prion strains.

SEED AMPLIFICATION ASSAYS FOR SYNUCLEINOPATHIES
α-Synuclein Real-Time Quaking-Induced Conversion and Protein Misfolding Cyclic Amplification

To provide molecular diagnoses of PD and dementia with Lewy bodies (DLB) and multiple system atrophy (MSA), several laboratories have now developed RT-QuIC–like assays for pathologic forms of α-synuclein (αSyn[D]), called αSyn RT-QuIC[58–63] or αSyn-PMCA.[64] These assays can have unprecedented sensitivity for αSyn[D] down into the low femtogram range and detect up to 10^8-fold dilutions of patients' brain tissue. When applied to CSF specimens collected from living patients, the diagnostic sensitivities for PD and DLB have ranged from 88% to 96% and specificities from 82% to 100%.[58,60,63–65] Blinded comparisons of the performance of 2 of these assays on a large set of patients with PD and healthy controls revealed a high degree of concordance in diagnostic performance.[65] Although the earlier assays took 5 to

13 days, newer permutations take 1 to 2 days[60] or 3 days[63] with comparable diagnostic performance and the ability to detect αSyn[D] seeds in CSF collected early in the clinical course of PD. Moreover, a recent study by Rossi and colleagues extensively validated a rapid αSyn RT-QuIC assay for Lewy body-associated α-synucleinopathies, e.g. Parkinson's disease and dementia with Lewy bodies.[66] Importantly, this study also detected αSyn[D] seeds in 18/18 isolated REM sleep behavior disorder and 26/28 pure autonomic failure cases prior to the appearance of parkinsonism or cognitive decline. Similarly rapid assays have been reported using postmortem submandibular gland tissue from PD and incidental Lewy body disease decedents, giving 100% sensitivity and 94% specificity for synucleinopathy.[62] αSyn[D] seeding activity can often be detected in nasal brushings from patients with synucleinopathy.[67] It is notable that studies have also reported evidence of strain-like differences between types of synucleinopathy-associated seeds.[60,61,68]

Although the multiple initial analyses of αSyn RT-QuIC and related assays have been encouraging, more extensive studies will be required to fully understand their diagnostic and prognostic utilities and the extent to which αSyn[D] seeding activities in accessible biospecimens might vary over time in individual patients. Such information will likely be important in understanding the extent to which the monitoring of αSyn[D] seeding activities might be helpful in setting up and assessing the progress of clinical trials of treatments designed to reduce αSyn[D] burden in the brain.

Human Embryonic Kidney Cell Bioassay for Multiple System Atrophy

Woerman and colleagues[69,70] expressed yellow fluorescent protein–tagged αSyn in human embryonic kidney (HEK) cells and found that phosphotungstic acid–precipitated extracts of brain homogenates from MSA decedents could be assayed on these cells 4 days after exposure by quantitating cells with fluorescent aggregates. The assay had an analytical sensitivity of 70 pg/mL, and revealed differences in regional distribution of αSyn seeding activity between patients with MSA. Interestingly, this assay was not sensitive to the αSyn seeds of PD cases.[69,70] The results provided evidence for the MSA and PD being distinct αSyn[D] prion strains.

HANdai Amyloid Burst Inducer Assay

Recently, an ultrasonication-based assay was described that uses the HANdai Amyloid Burst Inducer (HANABI) system to amplify αSyn[D].[71] Analogous to what is done in classic PMCA, the investigators applied ultrasonication to break up αSyn[D] oligomers in order to increase the nuclei from which the polymerization starts. The addition of αSyn preformed fibrils in artificial CSF enhanced the reaction speed in a dose-dependent fashion. Although ultrasonication provided faster reactions, it also increased the unseeded polymerization in negative control reactions. The analysis of human CSF from patients with PD and controls showed overlapping reaction kinetics, complicating the diagnostic sensitivity and specificity of this assay.

SEED AMPLIFICATION ASSAYS FOR TAUOPATHIES

Multiple neurodegenerative diseases involve the pathologic accumulation of tau filaments, including AD, chronic traumatic encephalopathy (CTE), progressive supranuclear palsy (PSP), corticobasal degeneration (CBD), frontotemporal dementia and parkinsonism 17 microtubule-associated protein tau (FTDP 17 *MAPT*), argyrophilic grain disease (AGD), and Pick disease (PiD). In adult humans, the alternative splicing of the *MAPT* gene gives rise to 6 tau isoforms. These isoforms differ from each other by the presence or absence of inserts near the N terminus and by the number of microtubule binding domains near the C terminus; that is, 3 (3R) or 4 (4R) isoforms. The tau pathologies of different diseases are characterized by the preferential deposition of 3R, 4R, or both 3R and 4R tau isoforms. For example, patients with AD and CTE accumulate roughly equivalent amounts of both 3R and 4R isoforms because all the isoforms contain the residues comprising the amyloid cores of the paired helical and straight tau filaments of these diseases.[72,73] Patients with PiD accumulate mainly 3R isoforms,[74,75] consistent with their compatibility with the distinct amyloid core of PiD filaments.[76] In contrast, patients with PSP, CBD, and FTDP 17 *MAPT* preferentially accumulate 4R isoforms, which, in the case of CBD, can again be rationalized by the core structure of the CBD-associated filaments.[77]

Tau Real-Time Quaking-Induced Conversion Assays

Initial studies by Margittai and colleagues showed that, in sonicated, multiwell plate–based reactions, synthetic fibrils formed with different 3R and 4R tau constructs had distinct seeding activities[78] and also that AD brain homogenates could seed the fibrilization of tau constructs faster than control homogenates.[79] Since then, ultrasensitive and selective tau RT-QuIC assays have been developed for disease-associated 3R, 4R, and 3R + 4R tau aggregates, and some subclasses thereof.[6,80–83] Tau RT-QuIC performance can be improved (ie, higher sensitivity can be achieved without compromising specificity) by systematic comparisons of conditions such as salts of the Hofmeister series.[82] These tau RT-QuIC assays can detect seeds in 10^8-fold to 10^{10}-fold dilutions of brain tissue, with orders of magnitude of selectivity for the types of tauopathy for which they were optimized. The optimization of each of these assays involved comparisons of various recombinant tau substrate constructs, cofactors, and other reaction components and conditions. Use of a 3R tau fragment (K19CFh) as a substrate first allowed the development of the 3R tau RT-QuIC assay, which specifically detects PiD seeds in brain tissue and postmortem CSF samples.[80] To detect AD and CTE tau filaments, a substrate (τ306) spanning the entire amyloid core of the associated filaments was then included in the reaction to allow the amplification of the seeds.[6] Seeds of multiple diseases with 4R tauopathy can be detected with the recently developed 4R Tau RT-QuIC.[81] This assay is the first tau RT-QuIC assay to allow detection of tau seeds in antemortem, as well as postmortem, CSF specimens. In addition, the authors more recently used another tau substrate (K12CFh) to develop a single tau RT-QuIC assay for the detection and discrimination of tau seeds of AD and PiD.[83] This assay simplifies the testing for these types of tau seeds and indicates that they differ in conformational templating activity. As with the prion and αSyn RT-QuIC assays, the ability to detect tau seeds in accessible diagnostic specimens will be important for antemortem diagnostic utility of tau RT-QuIC assays. However, at present, further research is necessary to better establish any such utility.

Another valuable feature of the 4R RT-QuIC assay is its ability to differentiate 3 classes of 4R tau seeds based on characteristics of the fibrillar reaction products, namely their relative enhancement of ThT fluorescence, and their β-sheet conformations as assessed by Fourier transform infrared (FTIR) spectroscopy: class A is represented by FTDP-17 with P301L *MAPT* mutation; class B includes the FTDP-17 with N279K mutation and CBD; and class C includes PSP.[81]

In applying tau RT-QuIC assays to biological specimens, it is important to bear in mind that various types of tau aggregates and seeding activities can be found at lower levels (usually by orders of magnitude) in brain tissue, at least of individuals without primary tauopathies.[6,80–83] Thus, the diagnostic specificities of these ultrasensitive assays when applied to biospecimens may depend on quantitative, as well as qualitative, differences in tau seeding activities.

Biosensor Cell Assays

A highly sensitive and specific biosensor cell seeding assay for tau seeds has also been developed[84,85] by exploiting the ability of tau aggregates to penetrate cells and induce the fibrillization of soluble endogenous tau.[86] Briefly, when engineered HEK293T cell lines expressing 3R or 4R tau constructs fused to fluorescent proteins were exposed to exogenous proteopathic tau, these protein aggregates penetrated the cells and seeded the polymerization of intracellular tau.[84] The intracellular protein aggregation was detected by fluorescence resonance energy transfer (FRET), which was measured by fluorescence microscopy or flow cytometry. The exposure of the cells to increasing amounts of recombinant tau fibrils resulted in the gain of FRET signal in a dose-dependent fashion. Moreover, the incubation of HEK293T cells expressing fluorescent 3R or 4R tau constructs, or both, with specific tauopathy brain lysates (eg, from AD, CTE, PSP, CBD, AGD) triggered the formation of tau inclusions, whereas no tau aggregation was induced by negative controls. This finding showed that the polymerization was promoted by aggregated tau and not by other protein aggregates. Comparison of tau seeds from multiple sources showed them to behave like different strains by inducing characteristic intracellular inclusions that could be faithfully propagated through many in vitro passages and then on inoculation into transgenic mice.[87] To compare the sensitivity of this technique with histology (the gold standard postmortem method to diagnose AD[88]), a time-course analysis in a tauopathy mouse model was performed. Tau seeding activity preceded histopathologic detection by more than 4 weeks. Although these experimental systems have revealed much about the prion-like propagation and strain-dependent seeding capacity of tau aggregates, the practicality of these cellular models for routine clinical diagnostic purposes in clinical practice may be limited by the need for tissue cultures and either immunostaining or flow cytometry.

β-AMYLOID SEED AGGREGATION ASSAYS
Kinetic Aggregation Assay

In addition to the aforementioned neurofibrillary tangles of tau, amyloid plaques of the β-amyloid (Aβ) peptide are major lesions found in brains from patients with AD.[89] To detect Aβ aggregates, Kelly and colleagues developed a seeded polymerization-based assay.[90] In this kinetic aggregation assay, Aβ aggregates from mammalian cell culture media, Caenorhabditis elegans lysates, and AD mouse brain homogenates seeded the fibrillization of monomeric $A\beta_{1-40}$ peptide, in a cell-free reaction containing ThT to monitor fibril formation over time. The amount of Aβ amyloid fibrils in the sample was proportional to the half-time of the growth phase (t50). To prove the specificity of this assay, experiments with αSyn aggregates were also conducted and differences in the kinetic reactions were observed, with reactions seeded with 4.3-μg/mL $A\beta_{1-40}$ fibrils showing a t50 of ~5 hours, whereas 14.5-μg/mL α-synuclein fibrils yielded a ~9-hour t50. The investigators stated that this selectivity is needed to allow the quantification of Aβ amyloid fibrils in tissues that can potentially contain other amyloid seeds; however, human biological specimens from patients with different neurodegenerative disorders were not assessed by this assay in order to prove its specificity.

β-Amyloid Protein Misfolding Cyclic Amplification

Continuing along these lines, Soto and colleagues developed an assay called Aβ-PMCA, which detects misfolded Aβ oligomers down to as little as 3 fmol in a multiwell plate–based assay with ThT readout as in RT-QuIC assays.[91] Application of Aβ-PMCA to CSF specimens from patients with and without AD provided discrimination between the 2 sets with 90% sensitivity and 92% specificity. Because it is well known that cognitively normal or other patients without AD can have some Aβ deposits in their brain tissue, the specificity of the Aβ-PMCA presumably depends on disease-dependent differences in concentration of Aβ seeds in the CSF. Seed concentration is typically inversely correlated with lag time in seeded protein polymerization reactions, which likely explains the shorter lag phases that were observed with CSF samples from patients with AD. This assay promises to provide a useful complement to the AD tau RT-QuIC assay described earlier in measuring the key pathologic protein aggregates of AD.

HUNTINGTON DISEASE SEED AMPLIFICATION ASSAY

The applicability of an ASA of postmortem brain extracts from human patients with Huntington diseases, and transgenic mice models thereof, was reported by Gupta and coworkers.[92] Misfolded huntingtin partially purified from the diseased brains induced amyloid formation of a largely polyglutamine substrate more rapidly than extracts from negative control brains. Although this assay is inhibited by components of crude brain tissue, hence the need for partial purification of the seeds from brain, it serves as a prototypic test for pathologic forms of huntingtin.

SUMMARY

Continuing work by many laboratories is yielding a growing panel of ultrasensitive assays for the various misfolded self-propagating protein aggregates that cause many neurodegenerative diseases. These assays provide important tools for fundamental research into the pathogenesis of these diseases. Moreover, the ability to detect miniscule amounts of such proteopathic aggregates as biomarkers in accessible specimens is allowing more accurate molecular diagnoses of diseases that can otherwise be difficult to discriminate, especially early in pathogenesis when appropriately targeted treatments are more likely to be successful. Importantly, given the frequency with which patients with neurodegenerative disease have more than 1 type of aggregated protein in their central nervous systems, the high sensitivity of these assays allows detection of both primary and secondary proteopathies. Such testing should also facilitate the development of new therapies by allowing clearer identification of cases and controls for clinical trials, as well as the measurement of specific protein seeds as key etiologic biomarkers over the course of treatment.

ACKNOWLEDGMENTS

This work was supported by the Intramural Research Program of the NIAID (National Institute of Allergy and Infectious Diseases), United States. The authors thank Anita Mora for graphics assistance.

DISCLOSURE

B. Caughey is an inventor on patents or patent applications relating to prion, αSyn, and tau RT-QuIC assays. N.C. Ferreira has nothing to disclose.

REFERENCES

1. Caughey B, Lansbury PT. Protofibrils, pores, fibrils, and neurodegeneration: separating the responsible protein aggregates from the innocent bystanders. Annu Rev Neurosci 2003;26:267–98.

2. Chiti F, Dobson CM. Protein misfolding, amyloid formation, and human disease: a summary of progress over the last decade. Annu Rev Biochem 2017;109:27–68.
3. Silveira JR, Raymond GJ, Hughson AG, et al. The most infectious prion protein particles. Nature 2005;437(7056):257–61.
4. Diaz-Villanueva JF, Diaz-Molina R, Garcia-Gonzalez V. Protein folding and mechanisms of proteostasis. Int J Mol Sci 2015;16(8):17193–230.
5. Powers ET, Morimoto RI, Dillin A, et al. Biological and chemical approaches to diseases of proteostasis deficiency. Annu Rev Biochem 2009;78:959–91.
6. Kraus A, Saijo E, Metrick MAI, et al. Seeding selectivity and ultrasensitive detection of tau aggregate conformers of Alzheimer disease. Acta Neuropathol 2019; 137:585–98.
7. Saborio GP, Permanne B, Soto C. Sensitive detection of pathological prion protein by cyclic amplification of protein misfolding. Nature 2001;411(6839):810–3.
8. Atarashi R, Moore RA, Sim VL, et al. Ultrasensitive detection of scrapie prion protein using seeded conversion of recombinant prion protein. Nature Meth 2007; 4(8):645–50.
9. Colby DW, Zhang Q, Wang S, et al. Prion detection by an amyloid seeding assay. Proc Natl Acad Sci U S A 2007;104(52):20914–9.
10. Atarashi R, Satoh K, Sano K, et al. Ultrasensitive human prion detection in cerebrospinal fluid by real-time quaking-induced conversion. Nature Med 2011;17(2): 175–8.
11. Wilham JM, Orrú CD, Bessen RA, et al. Rapid end-point quantitation of prion seeding activity with sensitivity comparable to bioassays. PLoS Path 2010; 6(12):e1001217.
12. Atarashi R, Wilham JM, Christensen L, et al. Simplified ultrasensitive prion detection by recombinant PrP conversion with shaking. Nature Meth 2008;5(3):211–2.
13. Barria MA, Gonzalez-Romero D, Soto C. Cyclic amplification of prion protein misfolding. Methods Mol Biol 2012;849:199–212.
14. Caughey B, Orru CD, Groveman BR, et al. Amplified detection of prions and other amyloids by RT-QuIC in diagnostics and the evaluation of therapeutics and disinfectants. Prog Mol Biol Transl Sci 2017;150:375–88.
15. Green AJE, Zanusso G. Prion protein amplification techniques. Handb Clin Neurol 2018;153:357–70.
16. Jarrett JT, Lansbury PT Jr. Seeding "one-dimensional crystallization" of amyloid: a pathogenic mechanism in alzheimer's disease and scrapie? Cell 1993;73: 1055–8.
17. Saa P, Castilla J, Soto C. Ultra-efficient replication of infectious prions by automated protein misfolding cyclic amplification. J Biol Chem 2006;281(46): 35245–52.
18. Orru CD, Wilham JM, Raymond LD, et al. Prion disease blood test using immunoprecipitation and improved quaking-induced conversion. Mbio 2011;2(3): e00078-11.
19. Zanusso G, Monaco S, Pocchiari M, et al. Advanced tests for early and accurate diagnosis of Creutzfeldt-Jakob disease. Nat Rev Neurol 2016;12(6):325–33.
20. Schmitz M, Cramm M, Llorens F, et al. The real-time quaking-induced conversion assay for detection of human prion disease and study of other protein misfolding diseases. Nature Protoc 2016;11(11):2233–42.
21. Bongianni M, Orrù CD, Groveman BR, et al. Diagnosis of human prion disease using real-time quaking-induced conversion testing of olfactory mucosa and cerebrospinal fluid samples. JAMA Neurol 2017;74(2):1–8.

22. Kocisko DA, Come JH, Priola SA, et al. Cell-free formation of protease-resistant prion protein. Nature 1994;370:471–4.
23. Kocisko DA, Priola SA, Raymond GJ, et al. Species specificity in the cell-free conversion of prion protein to protease-resistant forms: a model for the scrapie species barrier. Proc Natl Acad Sci U S A 1995;92:3923–7.
24. Bessen RA, Kocisko DA, Raymond GJ, et al. Nongenetic propagation of strain-specific phenotypes of scrapie prion protein. Nature 1995;375:698–700.
25. Bossers A, Belt PBGM, Raymond GJ, et al. Scrapie susceptibility-linked polymorphisms modulate the *in vitro* conversion of sheep prion protein to protease-resistant forms. Proc Natl Acad Sci USA 1997;94:4931–6.
26. Raymond GJ, Hope J, Kocisko DA, et al. Molecular assessment of the transmissibilities of BSE and scrapie to humans. Nature 1997;388:285–8.
27. Raymond GJ, Bossers A, Raymond LD, et al. Evidence of a molecular barrier limiting susceptibility of humans, cattle and sheep to chronic wasting disease. EMBO J 2000;19:4425–30.
28. Castilla J, Saa P, Hetz C, et al. In vitro generation of infectious scrapie prions. Cell 2005;121(2):195–206.
29. Castilla J, Morales R, Saa P, et al. Cell-free propagation of prion strains. EMBO J 2008;27(19):2557–66.
30. Castilla J, Saa P, Soto C. Detection of prions in blood. Nature Med 2005;11(9):982–5.
31. Soto C, Anderes L, Suardi S, et al. Pre-symptomatic detection of prions by cyclic amplification of protein misfolding. FEBS Lett 2005;579(3):638–42.
32. Gonzalez-Romero D, Barria MA, Leon P, et al. Detection of infectious prions in urine. FEBS Lett 2008;582(21–22):3161–6.
33. Moda F, Gambetti P, Notari S, et al. Prions in the urine of patients with variant Creutzfeldt-Jakob disease. N Engl J Med 2014;371(6):530–9.
34. Orru CD, Groveman BR, Raymond LD, et al. Bank vole prion protein as an apparently universal substrate for RT-QuIC-based detection and discrimination of prion strains. PLoS Path 2015;11(6):e1004983.
35. Caughey B, Orru CD, Groveman BR, et al. Detection and diagnosis of prion diseases using RT-QuIC: an update. In: Liberski P, editor. Prions diseases, Vol. 129. Basel (Switzerland): Springer Science+Business Media; 2017. p. 173–81.
36. Haley NJ, Richt JA, Davenport KA, et al. Design, implementation, and interpretation of amplification studies for prion detection. Prion 2018;12(2):73–82.
37. Orrú CD, Wilham JM, Hughson AG, et al. Human variant Creutzfeldt-Jakob disease and sheep scrapie PrP(res) detection using seeded conversion of recombinant prion protein. Protein Eng Des Sel 2009;22(8):515–21.
38. Wang Z, Manca M, Foutz A, et al. Early preclinical detection of prions in the skin of prion-infected animals. Nature Commun 2019;10(1):247.
39. McGuire LI, Peden AH, Orru CD, et al. RT-QuIC analysis of cerebrospinal fluid in sporadic Creutzfeldt-Jakob disease. Ann Neurol 2012;72(2):278–85.
40. Franceschini A, Baiardi S, Hughson AG, et al. High diagnostic value of second generation CSF RT-QuIC across the wide spectrum of CJD prions. Sci Rep 2017;7(1):10655.
41. Orru CD, Groveman BR, Hughson AG, et al. Rapid and sensitive RT-QuIC detection of human Creutzfeldt-Jakob disease using cerebrospinal fluid. MBio 2015;6(1) [pii:e02451-14].
42. Henderson DM, Denkers ND, Hoover CE, et al. Longitudinal detection of prion shedding in saliva and urine by chronic wasting disease-infected deer by real-time quaking-induced conversion. J Virol 2015;89(18):9338–47.

43. Orru CD, Yuan J, Appleby BS, et al. Prion seeding activity and infectivity in skin samples from patients with sporadic Creutzfeldt-Jakob disease. Sci Transl Med 2017;9(417) [pii:eaam7785].

44. Cheng YC, Hannaoui S, John TR, et al. Real-time quaking-induced conversion assay for detection of CWD prions in fecal material. J Vis Exp 2017;127.

45. Davenport KA, Mosher BA, Brost BM, et al. Assessment of chronic wasting disease prion shedding in deer saliva with occupancy modeling. J Clin Microbiol 2018;56(1) [pii:e01243-17].

46. Groveman BR, Orru CD, Hughson AG, et al. Extended and direct evaluation of RT-QuIC assays for Creutzfeldt-Jakob disease diagnosis. Ann Clin Transl Neurol 2017;4(2):139–44.

47. Foutz A, Appleby BS, Hamlin C, et al. Diagnostic and prognostic value of human prion detection in cerebrospinal fluid. Ann Neurol 2017;81(1):79–92.

48. Centers for Disease Control and Prevention. CDC's diagnostic criteria for Creutzfeldt-Jakob disease (CJD). 2018. Available at: https://www.cdc.gov/prions/cjd/diagnostic-criteria.html.

49. National CJD research and Surveillance Unit. Sporadic CJD diagnostic criteria. Available at: https://www.cjd.ed.ac.uk/sites/default/files/criteria_0.pdf.

50. Orru CD, Soldau K, Cordano C, et al. Prion seeds distribute throughout the eyes of sporadic creutzfeldt-jakob disease patients. MBio 2018;9(6).

51. Raymond, B. Race, C.D. Orru, et al., Transmission of CJD from nasal brushings but not spinal fluid or RT-QuIC products, Ann Clin Transl Neurol (in press).

52. Saijo E, Groveman BR, Kraus A, et al. Ultrasensitive RT-QuIC seed amplification assays for disease-associated tau, alpha-synuclein, and prion aggregates. Methods Mol Biol 2019;1873:19–37.

53. Klohn PC, Stoltze L, Flechsig E, et al. A quantitative, highly sensitive cell-based infectivity assay for mouse scrapie prions. Proc Natl Acad Sci U S A 2003; 100(20):11666–71.

54. Mahal SP, Demczyk CA, Smith EW Jr, et al. Assaying prions in cell culture: the standard scrapie cell assay (SSCA) and the scrapie cell assay in end point format (SCEPA). Methods Mol Biol 2008;459:49–68.

55. Schmidt C, Fizet J, Properzi F, et al. A systematic investigation of production of synthetic prions from recombinant prion protein. Open Biol 2015;5(12):150165.

56. van der Merwe J, Aiken J, Westaway D, et al. The standard scrapie cell assay: development, utility and prospects. Viruses 2015;7(1):180–98.

57. Sarell CJ, Quarterman E, Yip DC, et al. Soluble Abeta aggregates can inhibit prion propagation. Open Biol 2017;7(11).

58. Fairfoul G, McGuire LI, Pal S, et al. Alpha-synuclein RT-QuIC in the CSF of patients with alpha-synucleinopathies. Ann Clin Transl Neurol 2016;3(10):812–8.

59. Sano K, Atarashi R, Satoh K, et al. Prion-like seeding of misfolded alpha-synuclein in the brains of dementia with lewy body patients in RT-QUIC. Mol Neurobiol 2018;55(5):3916–30.

60. Groveman BR, Orru CD, Hughson AG, et al. Rapid and ultra-sensitive quantitation of disease-associated alpha-synuclein seeds in brain and cerebrospinal fluid by alphaSyn RT-QuIC. Acta Neuropathol Commun 2018;6(1):7.

61. Candelise N, Schmitz M, Llorens F, et al. Seeding variability of different alpha synuclein strains in synucleinopathies. Ann Neurol 2019;85(5):691–703.

62. Manne S, Kondru N, Jin H, et al. alpha-Synuclein real-time quaking-induced conversion in the submandibular glands of Parkinson's disease patients. Mov Disord 2020;35(2):268–78.

63. Bongianni M, Ladogana A, Capaldi S, et al. alpha-Synuclein RT-QuIC assay in cerebrospinal fluid of patients with dementia with Lewy bodies. Ann Clin Transl Neurol 2019;6(10):2120–6.
64. Shahnawaz M, Tokuda T, Waragai M, et al. Development of a biochemical diagnosis of Parkinson disease by detection of alpha-synuclein misfolded aggregates in cerebrospinal fluid. JAMA Neurol 2017;74(2):163–72.
65. Kang UJ, Boehme AK, Fairfoul G, et al. Comparative study of cerebrospinal fluid alpha-synuclein seeding aggregation assays for diagnosis of Parkinson's disease. Mov Disord 2019;34(4):536–44.
66. Rossi M, Candelise N, Baiardi S, et al., Ultrasensitive RT-QuIC assay with high sensitivity and specificity for Lewy body associated synucleinopathies. Acta Neuropathol 2020. doi:10.1007/s00401-020-02160-8. [Online ahead of print].
67. De Luca CMG, Elia AE, Portaleone SM, et al. Efficient RT-QuIC seeding activity for alpha-synuclein in olfactory mucosa samples of patients with Parkinson's disease and multiple system atrophy. Transl Neurodegener 2019;8:24.
68. Shahnawaz M, Mukherjee A, Pritzkow S, et al. Discriminating α-synuclein strains in Parkinson's disease and multiple system atrophy. Nature 2020;578(7794): 273–7.
69. Woerman AL, Stohr J, Aoyagi A, et al. Propagation of prions causing synucleinopathies in cultured cells. Proc Natl Acad Sci U S A 2015;112(35):E4949–58.
70. Prusiner SB, Woerman AL, Mordes DA, et al. Evidence for alpha-synuclein prions causing multiple system atrophy in humans with parkinsonism. Proc Natl Acad Sci U S A 2015;112(38):E5308–17.
71. Kakuda K, Ikenaka K, Araki K, et al. Ultrasonication-based rapid amplification of alpha-synuclein aggregates in cerebrospinal fluid. Sci Rep 2019;9(1):6001.
72. Fitzpatrick AWP, Falcon B, He S, et al. Cryo-EM structures of tau filaments from Alzheimer's disease. Nature 2017;547(7662):185–90.
73. Falcon B, Zivanov J, Zhang W, et al. Novel tau filament fold in chronic traumatic encephalopathy encloses hydrophobic molecules. Nature 2019;568(7752): 420–3.
74. Arai T, Ikeda K, Akiyama H, et al. Different immunoreactivities of the microtubule-binding region of tau and its molecular basis in brains from patients with Alzheimer's disease, Pick's disease, progressive supranuclear palsy and corticobasal degeneration. Acta Neuropathol 2003;105(5):489–98.
75. Irwin DJ, Brettschneider J, McMillan CT, et al. Deep clinical and neuropathological phenotyping of Pick disease. Ann Neurol 2016;79(2):272–87.
76. Falcon B, Zhang W, Murzin AG, et al. Structures of filaments from Pick's disease reveal a novel tau protein fold. Nature 2018;561(7721):137–40.
77. Zhang K, Tarutani A, Newell KL, et al. Novel tau filament fold in corticobasal degeneration, a four-repeat tauopathy. bioRxiv 2020;580(7802):283–7.
78. Dinkel PD, Siddiqua A, Huynh H, et al. Variations in filament conformation dictate seeding barrier between three- and four-repeat tau. Biochemistry 2011;50(20): 4330–6.
79. Meyer V, Dinkel PD, Rickman Hager E, et al. Amplification of Tau fibrils from minute quantities of seeds. Biochem 2014;53(36):5804–9.
80. Saijo E, Ghetti B, Zanusso G, et al. Ultrasensitive and selective detection of 3-repeat tau seeding activity in Pick disease brain and cerebrospinal fluid. Acta Neuropathol 2017;133(5):751–65.
81. Saijo E, Metrick MA 2nd, Koga S, et al. 4-Repeat tau seeds and templating subtypes as brain and CSF biomarkers of frontotemporal lobar degeneration. Acta Neuropathol 2020;139:63–77.

82. Metrick MA 2nd, do Carmo Ferreira N, Saijo E, et al. Million-fold sensitivity enhancement in proteopathic seed amplification assays for biospecimens by Hofmeister ion comparisons. Proc Natl Acad Sci U S A 2019;116(46):23029–39.

83. Metrick MAI, Ferreira NC, Saijo E, et al. A single ultrasensitive assay for detection and discrimination of tau aggregates of Alzheimer and Pick diseases. Acta Neuropathol Commun 2020;8(1):22.

84. Holmes BB, Furman JL, Mahan TE, et al. Proteopathic tau seeding predicts tauopathy in vivo. Proc Natl Acad Sci U S A 2014;111(41):E4376–85.

85. Woerman AL, Aoyagi A, Patel S, et al. Tau prions from Alzheimer's disease and chronic traumatic encephalopathy patients propagate in cultured cells. Proc Natl Acad Sci U S A 2016;113(50):E8187–96.

86. Guo JL, Lee VM. Seeding of normal Tau by pathological Tau conformers drives pathogenesis of Alzheimer-like tangles. J Biol Chem 2011;286(17):15317–31.

87. Kaufman SK, Sanders DW, Thomas TL, et al. Tau prion strains dictate patterns of cell pathology, progression rate, and regional vulnerability in vivo. Neuron 2016; 92(4):796–812.

88. Montine TJ, Phelps CH, Beach TG, et al. National Institute on Aging-Alzheimer's Association guidelines for the neuropathologic assessment of Alzheimer's disease: a practical approach. Acta Neuropathol 2012;123(1):1–11.

89. Reitz C, Mayeux R. Alzheimer disease: epidemiology, diagnostic criteria, risk factors and biomarkers. Biochem Pharmacol 2014;88(4):640–51.

90. Du D, Murray AN, Cohen E, et al. A kinetic aggregation assay allowing selective and sensitive amyloid-beta quantification in cells and tissues. Biochem 2011; 50(10):1607–17.

91. Salvadores N, Shahnawaz M, Scarpini E, et al. Detection of misfolded Abeta oligomers for sensitive biochemical diagnosis of Alzheimer's disease. Cell Rep 2014; 7(1):261–8.

92. Gupta S, Jie S, Colby DW. Protein misfolding detected early in pathogenesis of transgenic mouse model of Huntington disease using amyloid seeding assay. J Biol Chem 2012;287(13):9982–9.

Genetic Testing for Amyotrophic Lateral Sclerosis and Frontotemporal Dementia: Impact on Clinical Management

Jennifer Roggenbuck, MS, CGC[a],*, Jamie C. Fong, MS, CGC[b]

KEYWORDS

• ALS • FTD • *C9orf72* • Genetic testing • Genetic counseling

KEY POINTS

• Genetic testing is an increasingly important component in the management of amyotrophic lateral sclerosis (ALS) and frontotemporal dementia (FTD).
• A genetic cause may be identified in both familial and sporadic cases of ALS and FTD.
• All persons with ALS or FTD should be offered screening for the *C9orf72* repeat expansion; those with a family history of either condition or early onset of symptoms should be offered comprehensive multigene panel testing as a second step.
• Pretest and posttest counseling should emphasize the limitations and potential implications of testing.

INTRODUCTION

Ten years ago, commercial genetic testing for amyotrophic lateral sclerosis (ALS) was limited to *SOD1* sequencing, while only *MAPT* and *GRN* sequencing was available for frontotemporal dementia (FTD). Recent years have brought rapid progress in the discovery of genes associated with ALS and FTD, and a growing appreciation of the genetic component of both familial and sporadic disease. Commercial laboratories currently offer an array of multigene ALS, FTD, and combined ALS-FTD panels, assays for the *C9orf72* expansion, and whole-exome sequencing. The identification of a genetic cause now opens the door to a new era of genetic medicine for affected persons and their family members. As gene-targeted therapies move through the clinical trial pipeline, there is a need to prepare clinicians and laboratories to facilitate genetic diagnosis in ALS and FTD.

[a] Division of Human Genetics, Department of Neurology, The Ohio State University, 2012 Kenny Road, Columbus, OH 43221, USA; [b] Department of Molecular and Human Genetics, Baylor College of Medicine, One Baylor Plaza, MS: BCM115, Houston, TX 77030, USA
* Corresponding author.
E-mail address: jennifer.roggenbuck@osumc.edu

Clin Lab Med 40 (2020) 271–287
https://doi.org/10.1016/j.cll.2020.05.002
0272-2712/20/© 2020 Elsevier Inc. All rights reserved.

Genetics of Amyotrophic Lateral Sclerosis and Frontotemporal Dementia

- *C9orf72* is the most common known genetic cause of ALS, FTD, and ALS-FTD in persons of European descent.
- Most pathogenic variants in ALS and FTD genes are dominantly transmitted with variable and age-related penetrance.
- Symptoms, age of onset, and disease progression show significant intrafamilial and interfamilial variability.
- Genetic cause is more likely to be identified in patients with familial disease, but can also be found in sporadic cases.

ALS and FTD are adult-onset neurodegenerative disorders that share important clinical and pathologic features. ALS is characterized by loss of upper and lower motor neurons, progressive paralysis, and death within an average of 2 to 5 years after symptom onset. Diagnosis is made via clinical examination, electrodiagnostic testing, and exclusion of other diseases with similar symptoms. Treatment is palliative, and the only approved medical therapies include riluzole, which slows progression and prolongs survival by an average of 3 months,[1] and edaravone, which improves mobility in some patients.[2] FTD is a progressive disorder of behavior and language with insidious onset in middle to late adulthood associated with degeneration of the frontal and temporal brain lobes. Behavior variant FTD (bvFTD) comprises 1 subtype, and nonfluent variant primary progressive aphasia (nfvPPA) and semantic variant primary progressive aphasia (svPPA) comprise the 2 language subtypes. The 3 subtypes of FTD have overlapping features and are delineated by the behavior or language deficits that are the first persistent and predominant symptom in the course of illness. Postmortem analysis of brain tissue is the gold standard for diagnosis of FTD. However, in vivo diagnosis can be made with varied degrees of confidence by clinical examination, neuropsychological testing, and neuroimaging. There are no Food and Drug Administration–approved therapies for FTD; treatment is based on managing select behaviors nonpharmacologically and pharmacologically. For example, compulsive behaviors, disinhibition, and dysregulated eating may respond to selective serotonin reuptake inhibitors.[3]

Overlapping clinical, pathologic, and genetic features of ALS and FTD have long been recognized.[4] Approximately half of patients with ALS have cognitive impairment[5–7]: 5% to 15% meet criteria for FTD, and 35% have mild to moderate cognitive changes.[8] The hallmark ALS pathologic condition of TDP-43-positive neuronal cytoplasmic inclusions is found in 98% of ALS cases.[9] Although FTD has more neuropathologic heterogeneity than ALS, half of all FTD patients have tau-negative, TDP-43-positive cytoplasmic inclusions, referred to as FTLD-TDP. Furthermore, motor neuron pathology is found in most cases of FTLD-TDP even in the absence of clinical signs of ALS.[10] Pathogenic variants in many genes can cause ALS, FTD, or ALS-FTD. A hexanucleotide expansion in *C9orf72* is the most common genetic cause in cases of ALS, FTD, and combined ALS-FTD; multiple disease presentations are commonly observed in affected pedigrees.[11–13]

Cases of ALS and FTD are often classified as familial or sporadic, based on the presence or absence of a positive family history of a similar or related condition. However, sporadic and familial disease cannot be distinguished by clinical or pathologic features alone, and genetic cause may be found in both. One exception is *C9orf72*-mediated cases of FTD with or without ALS, which display unique neuropathologic findings upon postmortem analysis.[10,14] However, not all patients and their families have autopsy available to them, and some may decline autopsy. Approximately 10% of ALS cases and 40% of FTD cases are familial; a genetic cause may be identified in up to 70% of familial ALS cases and 10% of sporadic ALS cases, whereas a genetic cause may be identified in about 10% of familial FTD cases and 5% to 6% of sporadic FTD cases.[12,15,16] More than 30 genes have been identified that are implicated in ALS, FTD, or both.

Significant Amyotrophic Lateral Sclerosis and Frontotemporal Dementia Genes

Herein the authors outline the most prevalent ALS and FTD genes, in the order of their discovery, and highlight several genes associated with unique "crossover" motor neuron disease (MND) presentations (**Fig. 1**).

SOD1

In 1993, *SOD1* was the first gene identified to cause familial ALS (fALS),[17] and it is the second most common known cause of fALS in European populations after *C9orf72*. Notably, SOD1 is not associated with FTD. Persons with SOD1-related ALS have Lewy body-like inclusions that are positive for SOD1, ubiquitin, and phosphorylated neurofilaments, but negative for TDP-43 and FUS.[18] Pathogenic variants in *SOD1* are found in 12% of fALS and 1% to 2% of sALS cases, in European populations.[19] The frequency of pathogenic variants in SOD1 varies in different ethnogeographic populations, occurring, for example, in 38% of Irani familial ALS cases,[20] 30% of Chinese familial ALS cases,[21] and none of Irish familial ALS cases.[22] Specific variants are known to be associated with faster or slower disease progression: the Ala5Val variant, which accounts for a significant proportion of pathogenic *SOD1* variants in North America, causes a rapidly progressive course, whereas Gly37Arg, Gly41Asp, Glu100Lys, and Asp90Ala lead to a prolonged disease course. Most pathogenic variants in *SOD1* are transmitted in an autosomal dominant manner with variable and age-dependent penetrance. The Asp90Ala variant is known to cause recessive disease in Northern Scandinavia[23] and may be a lower-penetrance dominant variant in other populations.[22]

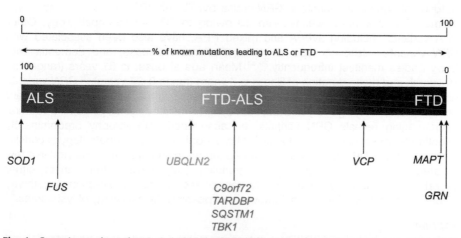

Fig. 1. Genetic overlap of ALS and FTD. (*Adapted from* Ling SC, Polymenidou M, Cleveland DW. Converging Mechanisms in ALS and FTD: Disrupted RNA and Protein Homeostasis. Neuron 79:3; p416-428.)

The first phase 1 trial of an SOD1 antisense oligonucleotide therapy, ASO 333611 (ISIS-SOD1$_{RX}$), was completed in 2012 (NCT01041222); a second-generation higher-dose ASO treatment (BIIB067, IONIS-SOD1$_{RX}$, NCT02623699) is currently being studied in a phase 1A/B randomized, placebo-controlled trial.[24]

MAPT

Autosomal dominant variants in *MAPT* cause bvFTD with or without parkinsonism, all owing to tau neuropathology. Select *MAPT* variants been associated with progressive supranuclear palsy (PSP). However, these PSP patients usually have an atypical or incomplete PSP syndrome, in addition to behavioral features consistent with bvFTD.[25–27] Mean age at onset is 49 years (range 17–82 years),[28] and mean duration of illness is 9 years (range 0–45 years). High penetrance (>95%) characterizes most *MAPT* variants, and a dementia-positive family history is almost always present.[29] Exceptions include variants located in exons 9 and 11 to 13, including the Arg406Trp variant. The Arg406Trp is pathogenic for FTLD, although carriers can present with varied clinical syndromes, including a clinical Alzheimer syndrome with late-onset frontal signs.[30–32] The Arg406Trp variant is usually associated with later-onset age and longer disease duration, compared with other *MAPT* variants.[33,34] Microscopic FTLD neuropathology is referred to as FTLD-tau. MND is not a common feature of *MAPT*-mediated disease.[35,36] *MAPT* encodes a scaffolding protein involved in the assembly and stabilization of microtubules.

CHMP2B

A heterozygous *CHMP2B* variant has been associated with bvFTD in 1 large Danish family[37] and 1 Belgian patient. *CHMP2B* variants are a rare cause of FTD.[38] Mean age at onset is 58 years (range 46–65 years).[38] MND has not been reported. Immunohistochemical analysis reveals inclusions that are positive for ubiquitin and negative for tau, TDP-43, and FUS. The pathologic condition is classified as FTLD-UPS (ubiquitin-proteasome system). CHMP2B encodes an endosomal sorting complex protein involved in vesicular trafficking in the endolysosomal pathway and the protein quality control process.[39,40]

GRN

Autosomal dominant variants in *GRN* cause bvFTD, nfvPPA, and corticobasal syndrome with or without parkinsonism, all owing to TDP-43 neuropathology. Other PPA variants, including svPPA and mixed PPA, have also been associated with *GRN* variants. Alzheimer-type dementia, Parkinson disease, and dementia with Lewy bodies manifest infrequently.[29,41] Mean age at onset is 61 years (range 25–90 years), and mean duration of illness is 7 years (range 0–27 years).[28] *GRN* variants display reduced penetrance, because 90% of people with a pathogenic GRN variant are symptomatic by age 70 years (50% are symptomatic by age 60 years).[42] Structural neuroimaging reveals GRN variants are associated with atrophy predominantly affecting temporal and parietal lobes.[43] Microscopic FTLD neuropathology is consistent with FTLD-TDP type A. MND is a rare phenotype and has been reported in a few isolated cases.[29,42] *GRN* encodes progranulin, a glycoprotein that can be either secreted and endocytosed or directly transported to the endolysosomal pathway where it regulates the formation, turnover, and possibly the exophagy of lysosomes.[42]

TARDBP

Pathogenic variants in *TARDBP* are autosomal dominant and cause both familial and sporadic ALS with varying degrees of cognitive deficits. Variants in *TARDBP* have also been observed in bvFTD patients with or without MND.[44–47] Patients who had cooccurring bvFTD and MND presented initially with a behavioral-cognitive syndrome and developed MND later in the illness course. A heterozygous Lys263Glu variant has also been identified in a patient with FTD, supranuclear gaze palsy, and chorea, but without MND.[48] Variants Ile383Val and Gly295Ser may present with semantic variant PPA, a language subtype of FTD. Microscopic ALS neuropathology features include TDP-43-positive cytoplasmic inclusions in glial cells of the spinal cord.[49,50] Microscopic neuropathology in patients with FTLD is consistent with FTLD-TDP, and although varied, may align best with FTLD-TDP type A.[51] TARDBP encodes the transactive DNA-binding protein 43, a RNA/DNA-binding protein thought to regulate multiple steps of RNA metabolism.[49]

FUS

Pathogenic variants in FUS most often present as MND and are found in about 5% of familial and less than 1% of sporadic ALS, including juvenile ALS.[52] Transmission is autosomal dominant. FTD associated with FUS variants is rare and has only been reported in a few families.[51,53] Referred to as ALS-FUS, microscopic ALS neuropathology is unique, featuring cytoplasmic inclusions positive for FUS and TDP-43. FTLD with underlying FUS neuropathology, referred to as FTLD-FUS, is well characterized. However, most cases of FTLD-FUS are not associated with FUS variants. Most patients with FTLD-FUS present with bvFTD and tend to be younger and have a more rapidly progressive clinical course. FUS encodes a nucleoprotein that functions in DNA and RNA metabolism, including DNA repair, and the regulation of transcription, RNA splicing, and export to the cytoplasm.[54]

VCP

Autosomal dominant variants in VCP cause a multisystem disorder characterized by adult-onset proximal and distal muscle weakness (90% of cases, clinically resembling a limb-girdle muscular dystrophy), early-onset Paget disease of the bone (51% of cases with osteolytic bone lesions), or FTD (32% of cases).[55,56] Because muscle weakness is the presenting symptom in more than half of people, inclusion body myopathy with Paget disease and frontotemporal dementia may frequently be seen in a neuromuscular clinic without its other syndromic features. Mean age at onset of muscle weakness is 45 years, whereas onset of associated dementia occurs later, with a mean age of 54 years.[55] Immunohistochemical analysis reveals a pathologic condition pattern (FTLD-TDP) characterized by extensive ubiquitin-positive intranuclear inclusions and dystrophic neurites in the temporal lobe. The inclusions are negative for tau, but positive for TDP-43.[56] This microscopic FTLD neuropathology is classified as FTLD-TDP type D, which is not seen in other genetic or sporadic FTD cases.[54] VCP encodes valosin-containing protein, a ubiquitously expressed multifunctional protein that has been implicated in multiple cellular functions ranging from organelle biogenesis to ubiquitin-dependent protein degradation.[56]

C9orf72

Expanded hexanucleotide (GGGGCC or G4C2) repeat variants in C9orf72 cause ALS, FTD, or ALS-FTD and are transmitted in an autosomal dominant fashion. In populations of European descent, pathogenic expansions have been observed in 37% of familial and 6% of sporadic cases of ALS, and in 18% of familial and 6% of sporadic cases of FTD.[12] Pathogenic expansions are found in 56% of European cases of familial FTD with motor neuron disease (FTD-MND), and 14% of cases of sporadic FTD-MND.[57] Mean age at onset is 58 years (range 20–91 years), and mean duration of illness is 6 years (range 0–36 years).[28,58,59] The 3 main phenotypes (ALS, FTD, and ALS-FTD) may occur in different individuals within a single family, but ALS-only or

FTD-only manifestations are also observed within single families. The most frequent C9orf72-associated FTD subtype is bvFTD.

Pathologically, patients with C9orf72-mediated disease display aggregation of TDP-43, accompanied by loss of nuclear TDP-43 within inclusion-bearing neurons.[14,59,60] The TDP-43-negative inclusions contain dipeptide-repeat (DPR) proteins generated by repeat-associated non-ATG (RAN) translation. DPR-positive pathologic condition is unique to the C9orf72 expansion. Microscopic FTLD neuropathology is consistent with FTLD-TDP type B.[10]

More than 95% of neurologically healthy people have 11 or fewer C9orf72 repeats.[21] The minimum repeat length threshold for pathogenicity has not been clearly established. An arbitrary cutoff of 30 repeats is used by most clinical laboratories. However, large expansions ranging from hundreds to thousands of repeats are most frequently observed in C9orf72-mediated ALS, FTD, or ALS-FTD.[14] Although early studies suggested the penetrance of C9orf72 repeat expansions approaches 100% by age 80, more recent data suggest that penetrance may be incomplete.[61,62] Further study is needed to understand the penetrance and disease expression in carriers of C9orf72 repeat expansions.

Phase 1 clinical trials targeting both the C9orf72 hexanucleotide repeat expansion and the toxic DPR produced via RAN translation are expected to open soon.[24]

SQSTM1

Variants in SQSTM1 cause Paget disease of the bone, as well as both familial and sporadic ALS; transmission is autosomal dominant. SQSTM1 variants have also been identified in patients presenting with bvFTD with or without MND.[43,63] The SQSTM1 gene encodes a scaffolding protein, which regulates various cellular processes, including NF-kB signaling and ubiquitin-mediated autophagy pathways.[64,65] Aberrant signaling arising from SQSTM1 gene variants likely disrupts immune homeostasis, which has previously been implicated in neurodegeneration, including in frontotemporal degeneration. Microscopic FTLD neuropathology is consistent with FTLD-TDP type B.[66]

UBQLN2

Four different variants in UBQLN2 have been reported in 4 unrelated families with X-linked ALS and X-linked ALS-dementia,[67] which included manifesting female heterozygotes. The dementia in one of the families was characterized as bvFTD, and in some individuals, the behavior-cognitive syndrome preceded MND. All individuals eventually developed MND. UBQLN2 variants are a rare cause of FTD. Microscopic neuropathology features include ubiquilin-positive and sparsely TDP-43-positive inclusions in neurons of the cortex and the spinal cord. UBQLN2 encodes ubiquilin 2, a member of the ubiquilin family of proteins that regulate the degradation of ubiquitinated proteins by the proteasome.[67–69]

TBK1

Loss-of function variants in TBK1 have been reported in people with FTD-ALS, FTD, and familial ALS; transmission is autosomal dominant. Microscopic FTLD neuropathology is consistent with either FTLD-TDP type A or B.[70–74] TBK1 encodes a signaling kinase, which is involved in regulation of NF-kB and autophagy pathways. TBK1 haploinsufficiency is the likely molecular genetic mechanism.[72]

ATXN2

Emerging data suggest that ATXN2 expansions (known to cause spinocerebellar ataxia type 2) may also cause ALS and may be as common in ALS cohorts as pathogenic variants in *TARDBP*; transmission is autosomal dominant.[75] Previously, intermediate-length expansions were reported to increase susceptibility to ALS. Cytoplasmic accumulation of ATXN2 can be seen in ALS cases with or without an *ATXN2* expansion. Cytoplasmic ATXN2 and TDP-43 aggregates have been observed in non-genetically mediated FTLD.[76] Variants in *ATXN2* are not known to cause FTD.

APPROACH TO GENETIC EVALUATION

Ten years ago, commercial genetic testing for ALS and FTD was limited to 3 genes (*SOD1* sequencing in ALS, and *MAPT* and *GRN* sequencing in FTD), and the etiologic link between these conditions was not fully recognized. Commercial laboratories now offer multigene ALS, FTD, and combined ALS-FTD panels, assays for the *C9orf72* and *ATXN2* expansions, and whole-exome sequencing. The utility of genetic testing as part of clinical management is valued by patients.[77,78] US care guidelines for ALS and FTD do not address the offer of genetic testing. Evidence suggests that there is a growing consensus to offer genetic testing to patients with familial disease, but there is no consistent approach to the offer of testing to the typical patient, who has apparently sporadic disease.[79,80] A recent survey of ALS clinicians revealed that 74% would be more likely to offer ALS genetic testing if testing guidelines were in place.[81] The authors outline an approach to the genetic evaluation of ALS and FTD that may be useful to pathologists, neurologists, genetic counselors, and other specialists who provide clinical genetic testing in this population.

THE IMPORTANCE OF FAMILY HISTORY

Although a genetic cause may be identified in cases of familial or sporadic ALS and FTD, family history information is nonetheless useful in guiding the approach to genetic testing and in providing pretest and posttest genetic counseling. A 3-generation pedigree, at minimum, should be obtained, documenting cases of ALS, FTD, other dementia, parkinsonism, movement disorders, frontotemporal or cerebellar degeneration, psychiatric disorders, and suicide. The family history should be reviewed for evidence of autosomal dominant transmission of these features, although incomplete penetrance, inaccurate or incomplete family history information, misdiagnosis, early death, and other factors may obscure a clear pattern. Although there is no universal definition for the definition of familial ALS or FTD, in practice most clinicians consider the presence of a first-, second-, or third-degree relative with the same disease presentation to represent familial disease.[82] This simple guideline notably may miss identification of families in which affected persons have different disease presentations, such as ALS and FTD, in families with a *C9orf72* expansion.[16] Pedigree classification tools may aid in the stratification of FTD patients who are likely to carry a pathogenic variant.[83] However, these tools have limited positive predictive value in patients whose family histories do not follow autosomal dominant inheritance.[84]

GENETIC TESTING

- All patients with ALS, FTD, or ALS-FTD should be offered genetic testing for the *C9orf72* repeat expansion.
- ALS, FTD, or ALS-FTD patients with a family history of ALS, FTD, or related condition should be offered multigene panel testing as a second step.
- Multigene panel testing should be considered as a second step in *C9orf72*-negative ALS, FTD, or ALS-FTD patients with a family history of unspecified dementia or other poorly defined cognitive-behavioral syndrome.

- *C9orf72*-negative ALS, FTD, or ALS-FTD patients with onset of symptoms less than 50 years of age should also be offered multigene panel testing.
- ALS, FTD, or ALS-FTD patients whose *C9orf72* and multigene panel testing is negative should be referred to a genetics professional to discuss further testing or research participation.

All patients of European descent who have ALS, FTD, or ALS-FTD, regardless of their family history, should be offered testing for the *C9orf72* expansion. The significant frequency of pathogenic expansions in sporadic disease (approximately 10% in ALS and 6% in FTD), the implications for risk assessment in relatives, and the availability of *C9orf72*-targeted therapeutic trials warrant this approach.[16,82] Studies have shown that limiting the offer of *C9orf72* expansion testing to ALS patients with a positive family history of ALS would mean missing 50% of *C9orf72* expansion carriers.[85] Although detection of the *C9orf72* expansion currently requires a special assay (a repeat-primed polymerase chain reaction [PCR] assay, which may be combined with a fluorescent amplicon length assay) this test is commercially available for as little as $250, yielding a low per-diagnosis cost.[82]

Patients with a family history of ALS, FTD, or ALS-FTD, who test negative for the *C9orf72* expansion, should be offered multigene panel testing. A wide variety of commercial ALS, FTD, and combined ALS-FTD multigene sequencing panels are available. Multigene panels, often referred to as next-generation sequencing or NGS panels, use massively parallel sequencing technology to achieve analysis of a few to hundreds of genes at once, in a cost- and time-effective manner. A combined ALS-FTD multigene panel should include the most prevalent ALS and FTD genes, including at minimum *SOD1, FUS, TARDBP, TBK1, VCP, SQSTM1, UBQLN2, GRN,* and *MAPT, APP, PSEN1, PSEN2.* Of note, genes *APP, PSEN1, PSEN2* are implicated in autosomal dominant early-onset Alzheimer disease (AD), which is distinct from FTD. Variants in AD-causing genes cause neither FTD nor ALS. However, the reasons for including AD-causing genes on an ALS-FTD gene panel are several-fold, as follows: (1) FTD is frequently misdiagnosed, and providers may have limited experience with the condition, as compared with AD, which is the most prevalent dementia; (2) there are reports of people with AD-causing variants presenting with a clinical FTD syndrome[86,87]; (3) autosomal dominant early-onset AD, occurring often in those under the age of 65 years, has different therapeutic research opportunities than does FTD, which occurs just as frequently as AD in people under the age of 65 years.[88] **Fig. 2** summarizes the testing schema outlined here.

Most commercial panels contain many more genes than the 12 proposed herein. Often dubbed "comprehensive" ALS-FTD panel tests, these large panels may include rare genes with acceptable evidence for pathogenicity, whereas some panels also include genes with insufficient evidence for pathogenic potential. Such panels may include genes that harbor variants causing clinical syndromes that resemble ALS, FTD, or both, but that feature neuropathology not completely consistent with FTLD or MND. In addition, laboratories vary in the depth of coverage provided; some can detect deletions and duplications using relative read depth.[89] Costs of multigene panels vary widely, and some commercial laboratories offer a steeply discounted patient-pay option. Laboratories offer *C9orf72* repeat expansion testing together with sequencing of other genes as a single test bundle of 2 separate test platforms (repeat-primed PCR and NGS) under a single test code for the convenience of the ordering provider. Some laboratories offer a multigene panel test but do not offer an assay for *C9orf72* expansions, the most common cause of genetic ALS, FTD, and ALS-FTD. There is no standard set of genes on any given commercial laboratory

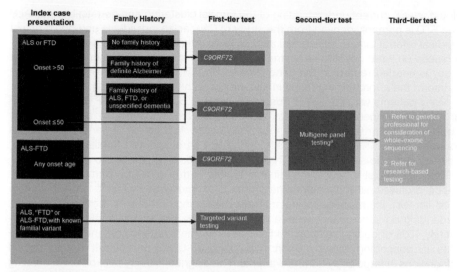

Fig. 2. Approach to the genetic evaluation of persons with ALS, FTD, or ALS-FTD. [a] Multi-gene panel testing should consist of, at minimum, *SOD1, FUS, TARDBP, TBK1, VCP, SQSTM1, UBQLN2, GRN,* and *MAPT, APP, PSEN1, PSEN2. ATNX2* repeat expansion testing should be ordered as a separate assay, concurrently or following multigene panel testing. (© The Ohio State University.)

test for ALS and FTD. Therefore, careful attention should be paid to the content of "comprehensive" ALS-FTD multigene tests, because their sensitivity and specificity will depend on which genes are included on the panel.

ALS and FTD patients who have an early onset of disease (onset of symptoms before or equal to 50 years of age), who test negative for the *C9orf72* expansion, should also be offered multigene panel testing. Although extensive data of the yield of genetic testing in this group are not available, 1 recent study found pathogenic or likely pathogenic variants in 18% of sporadic, early-onset ALS cases,[90] and such patients could harbor de novo pathogenic variants.[91]

Pathogenic expansions in *AXTN2*, which cause spinocerebellar ataxia type 2, have recently been identified as a cause of ALS and may be as common in ALS cohorts as pathogenic variants in *TARDBP*.[75] Detection of this repeat expansion requires a special assay, which should be offered for familial and early-onset ALS cases in whom no genetic cause is found after *C9orf72* repeat expansion and multigene panel testing. Pathogenic expansions in *ATXN2* are not a known cause of FTD.

The testing approach outlined here may be most applicable to patients of European ancestry. The variable ethnogeographic incidence of specific pathogenic variants (eg, the *C9orf72* expansion) may warrant population-specific testing approaches. For example, studies in Asian populations indicate that pathogenic variants in *SOD1* and *FUS* are more frequent causes of ALS than *C9orf72*.[21] Monogenic FTD is considered panethnic, but the variant frequency in causal genes varies worldwide from population to population. Monogenic FTD in South America appears to be due primarily to *C9orf72* expansions, whereas monogenic disease in Japan is attributed almost entirely to *MAPT* variants. Regional differences have emerged in the United States; for example, *MAPT* variants are most prevalent in FTD in the western United States, whereas central US states have a preponderance of patients with *GRN* variants.[28]

Nonetheless, current understanding of the familial clustering and genetic basis of ALS and FTD is primarily derived from the study of Caucasian individuals and could reflect medical referral biases, differential access to health care, as well as sociocultural differences on what constitutes normal behavior in instances of possible FTD. Further study is needed regarding the genetic basis of ALS and FTD in diverse populations to inform the approach to testing in all persons with these conditions.

Many patients with familial or possibly familial ALS, FTD, or ALS-FTD will not have an identifiable genetic cause despite comprehensive testing. In a recent study applying a similar testing schema in a clinic-based ALS cohort, a genetic cause was found in only 56% of fALS cases.[90] Patients with suspected familial disease may have a novel single-gene cause. These patients should be referred to a genetic counselor or geneticist to discuss additional testing and/or research participation. A genetics professional may determine whether exome sequencing is an appropriate third-tier test. Exome sequencing analyzes the coding portions of all genes. However, depending on sequencing depth and coverage, the platform can still miss approximately 10% of coding regions. Furthermore, exome sequencing cannot detect variants in noncoding regions or in mitochondrial DNA, nor can it detect repeat expansions or large copy number variants. The diagnostic utility of exome sequencing in this clinical patient population following negative C9orf72 and multigene panel testing is not known.[82]

LIMITATIONS AND CHALLENGES

Although a genetic cause is reported in 70% of fALS cases and 54% of familial FTD cases in research cohorts,[15] the yield of genetic testing in clinic populations may be lower. In particular, the incidence of pathogenic variants in genes other than C9orf72 may be lower in the clinic setting than expected from published research cohorts. Possible explanations for this discrepancy include the following: (1) the standards used in the interpretation of genetic variants identified in research may differ from those of the American College of Medical Genetics (ACMG)/American Molecular Pathologists (AMP), which are applied in clinical testing; (2) research cohorts may be enriched for fALS and familial FTD cases from "high-penetrance" pedigrees; (3) the geographic ancestry of the tested population may differ from that of research cohorts. Variants of uncertain significance (VUS), which do reach the ACMG/AMP standards for pathogenic classification, are commonly identified in clinical testing. However, such variants may be considered causative in research testing. ACMG/AMP criteria for variant pathogenicity rely on several lines of published evidence, including functional studies demonstrating a deleterious effect, and cosegregation with disease in multiple affected family members.[92] Functional studies are not available for many ALS and FTD genes, and segregation data are limited because affected relatives are not often available for testing because of limitations owing to advanced disease or death. Efforts are underway to revise ACMG/AMP criteria for ALS variant interpretation using disease specific and gene-specific data.[93]

In addition to the issues with result interpretation, there are also challenges with the technical aspects of testing. The accuracy of PCR-based C9orf72 assays has been questioned. Exact sizing of an expanded repeat is difficult because of its 100% GC content, its large size of 6 base pair repeat, somatic instability, and the repetitive nature of its flanking sequences. In a blinded study of commercial laboratories using PCR-based techniques, only 5/14 laboratories reported C9orf72 results in complete concordance with the reference Southern blot result, and both false negative and false positive results were identified.[93] A 10 base pair deletion adjacent to the repeat has been shown to interfere with detection of the expansion using PCR-based assays.[94] Despite the recommendation that Southern blot be used for clinical *C9orf72* testing, only 1 commercial laboratory in the United States currently offers this assay; another laboratory performs a 2-step protocol combining both a fluorescent amplicon length assay and a repeat-primed PCR that increases sensitivity and specificity in detecting expansions. Furthermore, the repeat size cutoffs for normal, intermediate, and expanded alleles vary; interpretations of intermediate results may also vary. There is currently no validated cutoff that differentiates between pathologic and nonpathologic alleles, but most patients with pathogenic expansions have hundreds to thousands of repeats.[95]

Data regarding small expansions between 30 and 100 repeats in size are lacking. There is evidence that a repeat size as short as 47 units in blood can present with ALS or FTD.[96] On the other hand, the identification of intermediate alleles in patients with ALS and FTD may be incidental. Furthermore, expansion sizes in blood may differ from those in relevant neural tissues because of somatic instability, further complicating result interpretation. There is no consensus regarding correlations between repeat size, quantified in blood or brain, and clinical variables. Laboratory test reports should ideally emphasize the clinicopathologic variability and age-dependent penetrance of pathologic expansions and include a statement that the pathogenicity of repeat sizes between 20 and 100 is unknown but likely increases with the size of the repeat.[95]

Variants of uncertain significance (VUS) are frequently identified in multigene panel testing,[95] including ALS and FTD panels. A recent survey of US commercial laboratories found that VUS rates on ALS multigene panels ranged from 12% to 30%, suggesting that many patients with ALS have received a VUS result. VUS outcomes present a challenge for clinicians and may be confusing to patients. Although rare variant burden may play a role in disease risk, VUS must be approached with caution in the clinical setting. Further data are needed regarding test methods and outcomes, including accuracy of current *C9orf72* assays, as well as guidance with VUS interpretation. False positive or negative results could have profound implications for patients and family members.[62,95]

THE IMPORTANCE OF A GENETIC DIAGNOSIS

Despite the challenges and limitations of current technology, genetic testing has the potential to empower persons and families affected by ALS and FTD. Many affected persons wish to know why they developed their condition, irrespective of their family history, and understanding the cause can bring a sense of accommodation and closure[16,77,82] as well as facilitate enrollment in gene-specific natural history studies. In some cases, a genetic diagnosis can provide valuable prognostic information, such as the likelihood of developing specific symptoms or expected rate of disease progression. Increasingly, persons with genetically characterized disease may be candidates for gene-targeted clinical trials, such as the current trial of BIIB067, an antisense oligonucleotide therapy for persons with *SOD1*-related ALS. Additional small molecule, virally- or antibody-mediated trials for other genetic forms of ALS and FTD are ongoing or imminent.[24]

A genetic diagnosis also has significant implications for family members, enabling specific risk assessment and providing the opportunity to undergo presymptomatic testing. At-risk individuals may wish to learn their genetic status to plan many aspects of their lives, including education, career, finances, insurance, disease surveillance, reproduction, and research participation. Furthermore, an affected family member's negative genetic testing, in the setting of sporadic disease with typical onset, may provide family members with reassurance that they have a low chance of developing disease.

Although genetic evaluation should be offered to every person with ALS or FTD, the decision to accept it remains a personal one, and some persons and families may struggle with this decision. In such cases or any case of genetic testing, a referral to a genetic counselor may be appropriate. Pretest genetic counseling will help individuals anticipate the impact of genetic testing in their personal and family context. Those who are cognitively impaired should be accompanied by a legal guardian or health care proxy. The limitations of genetic testing should be emphasized, including the following: (a) a negative result does not exclude a genetic basis or contribution to the condition; (b) the test may be uninformative if a variant of uncertain significance is identified; and (c) positive results do not uniformly allow prediction of penetrance or disease course. Families who are not ready to undergo genetic testing may consider DNA banking to permit future testing.[82]

SUMMARY

A growing appreciation of the genetic cause of both familial and sporadic ALS and FTD, the accessibility of commercial genetic testing, and the advent of gene-targeted clinical trials have ushered in a new era of genetic medicine for these neurodegenerative diseases. Genetic testing is now a vital component of disease management for both ALS and FTD. All affected persons should be offered screening for the C9orf72 repeat expansion; those at higher risk for a genetic cause should be offered multigene panel testing as a second step. Pretest and posttest counseling should highlight the limitations and potential implications of testing. With access to comprehensive genetic testing and counseling, persons and families with ALS and FTD can fully benefit from the remarkable advances in gene discovery in recent years.

ACKNOWLEDGEMENTS

We thank the Julie Bonasera Fund for ALS and Neuromuscular Diseases for support.

REFERENCES

1. Blasco H, Patin F, Andres CR, et al. Amyotrophic lateral sclerosis, 2016: existing therapies and the ongoing search for neuroprotection. Expert Opin Pharmacother 2016;17(12):1669–82.
2. Writing Group, Edaravone (MCI-186) ALS 19 Study Group. Safety and efficacy of edaravone in well defined patients with amyotrophic lateral sclerosis: a randomised, double-blind, placebo-controlled trial. Lancet Neurol 2017;16(7):505–12.
3. Rabinovici GD, Miller BL. Frontotemporal lobar degeneration: epidemiology, pathophysiology, diagnosis and management. CNS Drugs 2010;24(5):375–98.
4. Burrell JR, Halliday GM, Kril JJ, et al. The frontotemporal dementia-motor neuron disease continuum. Lancet 2016;388(10047):919–31.
5. Strong MJ, Lomen-Hoerth C, Caselli RJ, et al. Cognitive impairment, frontotemporal dementia, and the motor neuron diseases. Ann Neurol 2003;54(Suppl 5): S20–3.
6. Lomen-Hoerth C, Anderson T, Miller B. The overlap of amyotrophic lateral sclerosis and frontotemporal dementia. Neurology 2002;59(7):1077–9.
7. Lomen-Hoerth C, Murphy J, Langmore S, et al. Are amyotrophic lateral sclerosis patients cognitively normal? Neurology 2003;60(7):1094–7.
8. Tsermentseli S, Leigh PN, Goldstein LH. The anatomy of cognitive impairment in amyotrophic lateral sclerosis: more than frontal lobe dysfunction. Cortex 2012; 48(2):166–82.

9. Neumann M, Sampathu DM, Kwong LK, et al. Ubiquitinated TDP-43 in frontotemporal lobar degeneration and amyotrophic lateral sclerosis. Science 2006; 314(5796):130–3.

10. Mackenzie IRA, Neumann M. Molecular neuropathology of frontotemporal dementia: insights into disease mechanisms from postmortem studies. J Neurochem 2016;138(Suppl 1):54–70.

11. Renton AE, Majounie E, Waite A, et al. A hexanucleotide repeat expansion in C9ORF72 is the cause of chromosome 9p21-linked ALS-FTD. Neuron 2011; 72(2):257–68.

12. Majounie E, Renton AE, Mok K, et al. Frequency of the C9orf72 hexanucleotide repeat expansion in patients with amyotrophic lateral sclerosis and frontotemporal dementia: a cross-sectional study. Lancet Neurol 2012;11(4):323–30.

13. DeJesus-Hernandez M, Mackenzie IR, Boeve BF, et al. Expanded GGGGCC hexanucleotide repeat in noncoding region of C9ORF72 causes chromosome 9p-linked FTD and ALS. Neuron 2011;72(2):245–56.

14. Vatsavayai SC, Nana AL, Yokoyama JS, et al. C9orf72-FTD/ALS pathogenesis: evidence from human neuropathological studies. Acta Neuropathol 2019; 137(1):1–26.

15. Chia R, Chiò A, Traynor BJ. Novel genes associated with amyotrophic lateral sclerosis: diagnostic and clinical implications. Lancet Neurol 2018;17(1):94–102.

16. Turner MR, Al-Chalabi A, Chiò A, et al. Genetic screening in sporadic ALS and FTD. J Neurol Neurosurg Psychiatry 2017;88(12):1042–4.

17. Rosen DR, Siddique T, Patterson D, et al. Mutations in Cu/Zn superoxide dismutase gene are associated with familial amyotrophic lateral sclerosis. Nature 1993; 362(6415):59–62.

18. Saberi S, Stauffer JE, Schulte DJ, et al. Neuropathology of amyotrophic lateral sclerosis and its variants. Neurol Clin 2015;33(4):855–76.

19. Chiò A, Traynor BJ, Lombardo F, et al. Prevalence of SOD1 mutations in the Italian ALS population. Neurology 2008;70(7):533–7.

20. Alavi A, Nafissi S, Rohani M, et al. Genetic analysis and SOD1 mutation screening in Iranian amyotrophic lateral sclerosis patients. Neurobiol Aging 2013;34(5): 1516.e1-8.

21. Zou Z-Y, Zhou Z-R, Che C-H, et al. Genetic epidemiology of amyotrophic lateral sclerosis: a systematic review and meta-analysis. J Neurol Neurosurg Psychiatry 2017;88(7):540–9.

22. Kenna KP, McLaughlin RL, Byrne S, et al. Delineating the genetic heterogeneity of ALS using targeted high-throughput sequencing. J Med Genet 2013;50(11): 776–83.

23. Själander A, Beckman G, Deng H-X, et al. The D90A mutation results in a polymorphism of Cu, Zn superoxide dismutase that is prevalent in northern Sweden and Finland. Hum Mol Genet 1995;4(6):1105–8.

24. Ly CV, Miller TM. Emerging antisense oligonucleotide and viral therapies for amyotrophic lateral sclerosis. Curr Opin Neurol 2018;31(5):648–54.

25. Ogaki K, Li Y, Takanashi M, et al. Analyses of the MAPT, PGRN, and C9orf72 mutations in Japanese patients with FTLD, PSP, and CBS. Parkinsonism Relat Disord 2013;19(1):15–20.

26. Rohrer JD, Paviour D, Vandrovcova J, et al. Novel L284R MAPT mutation in a family with an autosomal dominant progressive supranuclear palsy syndrome. Neurodegener Dis 2011;8(3):149–52.

27. Spina S, Farlow MR, Unverzagt FW, et al. The tauopathy associated with muta-tion +3 in intron 10 of Tau: characterization of the MSTD family. Brain 2008; 131(Pt 1):72–89.

28. Moore KM, Nicholas J, Grossman M, et al. Age at symptom onset and death and disease duration in genetic frontotemporal dementia: an international retrospec-tive cohort study. Lancet Neurol 2019. https://doi.org/10.1016/S1474-4422(19) 30394-1.

29. Benussi L, Ghidoni R, Pegoiani E, et al. Progranulin Leu271LeufsX10 is one of the most common FTLD and CBS associated mutations worldwide. Neurobiol Dis 2009;33(3):379–85.

30. Lindquist SG, Holm IE, Schwartz M, et al. Alzheimer disease-like clinical pheno-type in a family with FTDP-17 caused by a MAPT R406W mutation. Eur J Neurol 2008;15(4):377–85.

31. Ikeuchi T, Kaneko H, Miyashita A, et al. Mutational analysis in early-onset familial dementia in the Japanese population. The role of PSEN1 and MAPT R406W mu-tations. Dement Geriatr Cogn Disord 2008;26(1):43–9.

32. Rademakers R, Dermaut B, Peeters K, et al. Tau (MAPT) mutation Arg406Trp pre-senting clinically with Alzheimer disease does not share a common founder in Western Europe. Hum Mutat 2003;22(5):409–11.

33. van Swieten JC, Stevens M, Rosso SM, et al. Phenotypic variation in hereditary frontotemporal dementia with tau mutations. Ann Neurol 1999;46(4):617–26.

34. Reed LA, Grabowski TJ, Schmidt ML, et al. Autosomal dominant dementia with widespread neurofibrillary tangles. Ann Neurol 1997;42(4):564–72.

35. Di Fonzo A, Ronchi D, Gallia F, et al. Lower motor neuron disease with respiratory failure caused by a novel MAPT mutation. Neurology 2014;82(22):1990–8.

36. Zarranz JJ, Ferrer I, Lezcano E, et al. A novel mutation (K317M) in the MAPT gene causes FTDP and motor neuron disease. Neurology 2005;64(9):1578–85.

37. Skibinski G, Parkinson NJ, Brown JM, et al. Mutations in the endosomal ESCRTIII-complex subunit CHMP2B in frontotemporal dementia. Nat Genet 2005;37(8): 806–8.

38. Ng AS, Rademakers R, Miller B. Frontotemporal dementia: a bridge between de-mentia and neuromuscular disease. Ann N Y Acad Sci 2015;1338(1):71–93.

39. Holm IE, Isaacs AM, Mackenzie IRA. Absence of FUS-immunoreactive pathology in frontotemporal dementia linked to chromosome 3 (FTD-3) caused by mutation in the CHMP2B gene. Acta Neuropathol 2009;118(5):719–20.

40. Mackenzie IRA, Neumann M, Cairns NJ, et al. Novel types of frontotemporal lobar degeneration: beyond tau and TDP-43. J Mol Neurosci 2011;45(3):402–8.

41. Wojtas A, Heggeli KA, Finch N, et al. C9ORF72 repeat expansions and other FTD gene mutations in a clinical AD patient series from Mayo Clinic. Am J Neurode-gener Dis 2012;1(1):107–18.

42. Gass J, Cannon A, Mackenzie IR, et al. Mutations in progranulin are a major cause of ubiquitin-positive frontotemporal lobar degeneration. Hum Mol Genet 2006;15(20):2988–3001.

43. Le Ber I, Camuzat A, Guerreiro R, et al. SQSTM1 mutations in French patients with frontotemporal dementia or frontotemporal dementia with amyotrophic lateral sclerosis. JAMA Neurol 2013;70(11):1403–10.

44. Chiang H-H, Andersen PM, Tysnes O-B, et al. Novel TARDBP mutations in Nordic ALS patients. J Hum Genet 2012;57(5):316–9.

45. Benajiba L, Le Ber I, Camuzat A, et al. TARDBP mutations in motoneuron disease with frontotemporal lobar degeneration. Ann Neurol 2009;65(4):470–3.

46. Floris G, Borghero G, Cannas A, et al. Clinical phenotypes and radiological findings in frontotemporal dementia related to TARDBP mutations. J Neurol 2015; 262(2):375–84.

47. Borroni B, Bonvicini C, Alberici A, et al. Mutation within TARDBP leads to frontotemporal dementia without motor neuron disease. Hum Mutat 2009;30(11): E974–83.

48. Kovacs GG, Murrell JR, Horvath S, et al. TARDBP variation associated with frontotemporal dementia, supranuclear gaze palsy, and chorea. Mov Disord 2009; 24(12):1843–7.

49. Gendron TF, Rademakers R, Petrucelli L. TARDBP mutation analysis in TDP-43 proteinopathies and deciphering the toxicity of mutant TDP-43. J Alzheimers Dis 2013;33(Suppl 1):S35–45.

50. Takeda T, Iijima M, Shimizu Y, et al. p.N345K mutation in TARDBP in a patient with familial amyotrophic lateral sclerosis: an autopsy case. Neuropathology 2019; 39(4):286–93.

51. Deng H, Gao K, Jankovic J. The role of FUS gene variants in neurodegenerative diseases. Nat Rev Neurol 2014;10(6):337–48.

52. Lattante S, Rouleau GA, Kabashi E. TARDBP and FUS mutations associated with amyotrophic lateral sclerosis: summary and update. Hum Mutat 2013;34(6): 812–26.

53. Yan J, Deng H-X, Siddique N, et al. Frameshift and novel mutations in FUS in familial amyotrophic lateral sclerosis and ALS/dementia. Neurology 2010;75(9): 807–14.

54. Hofmann JW, Seeley WW, Huang EJ. RNA binding proteins and the pathogenesis of frontotemporal lobar degeneration. Annu Rev Pathol 2019;14:469–95.

55. Weihl CC, Pestronk A, Kimonis VE. Valosin-containing protein disease: inclusion body myopathy with Paget's disease of the bone and fronto-temporal dementia. Neuromuscul Disord 2009;19(5):308–15.

56. Watts GDJ, Wymer J, Kovach MJ, et al. Inclusion body myopathy associated with Paget disease of bone and frontotemporal dementia is caused by mutant valosin-containing protein. Nat Genet 2004;36(4):377 81.

57. van der Zee J, Gijselinck I, Dillen L, et al. A pan-European study of the C9orf72 repeat associated with FTLD: geographic prevalence, genomic instability, and intermediate repeats. Hum Mutat 2013;34(2):363–73.

58. Boeve BF, Graff-Radford NR. Cognitive and behavioral features of c9FTD/ALS. Alzheimers Res Ther 2012;4(4):29.

59. Hsiung G-YR, DeJesus-Hernandez M, Feldman HH, et al. Clinical and pathological features of familial frontotemporal dementia caused by C9ORF72 mutation on chromosome 9p. Brain 2012;135(Pt 3):709–22.

60. Al-Sarraj S, King A, Troakes C, et al. p62 positive, TDP-43 negative, neuronal cytoplasmic and intranuclear inclusions in the cerebellum and hippocampus define the pathology of C9orf72-linked FTLD and MND/ALS. Acta Neuropathol 2011;122(6):691–702.

61. Murphy NA, Arthur KC, Tienari PJ, et al. Age-related penetrance of the C9orf72 repeat expansion. Sci Rep 2017;7. https://doi.org/10.1038/s41598-017-02364-1.

62. Crook A, McEwen A, Fifita JA, et al. The C9orf72 hexanucleotide repeat expansion presents a challenge for testing laboratories and genetic counseling. Amyotroph Lateral Scler Frontotemporal Degener 2019;20(5–6):310–6.

63. Rubino E, Rainero I, Chiò A, et al. SQSTM1 mutations in frontotemporal lobar degeneration and amyotrophic lateral sclerosis. Neurology 2012;79(15):1556–62.

64. Foster A, Scott D, Layfield R, et al. An FTLD-associated SQSTM1 variant impacts Nrf2 and NF-κB signalling and is associated with reduced phosphorylation of p62. Mol Cell Neurosci 2019;98:32–45.
65. Rea SL, Majcher V, Searle MS, et al. SQSTM1 mutations – bridging Paget disease of bone and ALS/FTLD. Exp Cell Res 2014;325(1):27–37.
66. Kovacs GG, van der Zee J, Hort J, et al. Clinicopathological description of two cases with SQSTM1 gene mutation associated with frontotemporal dementia. Neuropathology 2016;36(1):27–38.
67. Deng H-X, Chen W, Hong S-T, et al. Mutations in UBQLN2 cause dominant X-linked juvenile and adult-onset ALS and ALS/dementia. Nature 2011; 477(7363):211–5.
68. Fecto F, Siddique T. Making connections: pathology and genetics link amyotrophic lateral sclerosis with frontotemporal lobe dementia. J Mol Neurosci 2011; 45(3):663–75.
69. Williams JA, Thomas AM, Li G, et al. Tissue specific induction of p62/Sqstm1 by Farnesoid X receptor. PLoS One 2012;7(8). https://doi.org/10.1371/journal.pone.0043961.
70. Koriath CAM, Bocchetta M, Brotherhood E, et al. The clinical, neuroanatomical, and neuropathologic phenotype of TBK1-associated frontotemporal dementia: a longitudinal case report. Alzheimers Dement (Amst) 2017;6:75–81.
71. Cirulli ET, Lasseigne BN, Petrovski S, et al. Exome sequencing in amyotrophic lateral sclerosis identifies risk genes and pathways. Science 2015;347(6229): 1436–41.
72. Freischmidt A, Wieland T, Richter B, et al. Haploinsufficiency of TBK1 causes familial ALS and fronto-temporal dementia. Nat Neurosci 2015;18(5):631–6.
73. Gijselinck I, Van Mossevelde S, van der Zee J, et al. Loss of TBK1 is a frequent cause of frontotemporal dementia in a Belgian cohort. Neurology 2015;85(24): 2116–25.
74. Pottier C, Bieniek KF, Finch N, et al. Whole-genome sequencing reveals important role for TBK1 and OPTN mutations in frontotemporal lobar degeneration without motor neuron disease. Acta Neuropathol 2015;130(1):77–92.
75. Moreno C, Hoover B, Likanje M, et al. Pathogenic ATXN2 repeat expansions are as common as TARDBP mutations in large ALS cohorts. In: Northeast ALS Consortium Conference, October 4, 2019, Clearwater Beach, FL.
76. Elden AC, Kim H-J, Hart MP, et al. Ataxin-2 intermediate-length polyglutamine expansions are associated with increased risk for ALS. Nature 2010;466(7310): 1069–75.
77. Wagner KN, Nagaraja H, Allain DC, et al. Patients with amyotrophic lateral sclerosis have high interest in and limited access to genetic testing. J Genet Couns 2017;26(3):604–11.
78. Wagner KN, Nagaraja HN, Allain DC, et al. Patients with sporadic and familial amyotrophic lateral sclerosis found value in genetic testing. Mol Genet Genomic Med 2018;6(2):224–9.
79. Goldman JS, Van Deerlin VM. Alzheimer's disease and frontotemporal dementia: the current state of genetics and genetic testing since the advent of next-generation sequencing. Mol Diagn Ther 2018;22(5):505–13.
80. Vajda A, McLaughlin RL, Heverin M, et al. Genetic testing in ALS: a survey of current practices. Neurology 2017;88(10):991–9.
81. Klepek H, Nagaraja H, Goutman SA, et al. Lack of consensus in ALS genetic testing practices and divergent views between ALS clinicians and patients. Amyotroph Lateral Scler Frontotemporal Degener 2019;20(3–4):216–21.

82. Roggenbuck J, Quick A, Kolb SJ. Genetic testing and genetic counseling for amyotrophic lateral sclerosis: an update for clinicians. Genet Med 2017;19(3): 267–74.
83. Goldman JS, Farmer JM, Wood EM, et al. Comparison of family histories in FTLD subtypes and related tauopathies. Neurology 2005;65(11):1817–9.
84. Beck J, Rohrer JD, Campbell T, et al. A distinct clinical, neuropsychological and radiological phenotype is associated with progranulin gene mutations in a large UK series. Brain 2008;131(Pt 3):706–20.
85. Umoh ME, Fournier C, Li Y, et al. Comparative analysis of C9orf72 and sporadic disease in an ALS clinic population. Neurology 2016;87(10):1024–30.
86. Mahoney CJ, Downey LE, Beck J, et al. The presenilin 1 P264L mutation presenting as non-fluent/agrammatic primary progressive aphasia. J Alzheimers Dis 2013;36(2):239–43.
87. Riudavets MA, Bartoloni L, Troncoso JC, et al. Familial dementia with frontotemporal features associated with M146V presenilin-1 mutation. Brain Pathol 2013; 23(5):595–600.
88. Ratnavalli E, Brayne C, Dawson K, et al. The prevalence of frontotemporal dementia. Neurology 2002;58(11):1615–21.
89. Truty R, Patil N, Sankar R, et al. Possible precision medicine implications from genetic testing using combined detection of sequence and intragenic copy number variants in a large cohort with childhood epilepsy. Epilepsia Open 2019;4(3): 397–408.
90. Roggenbuck J, Palettas M, Vicini L, et al. Incidence of pathogenic, likely pathogenic, and uncertain ALS variants in a clinic cohort. Neurol Genet 2020;6(1). https://doi.org/10.1212/NXG.0000000000000390.
91. Hübers A, Just W, Rosenbohm A, et al. De novo FUS mutations are the most frequent genetic cause in early-onset German ALS patients. Neurobiol Aging 2015;36(11):3117.e1–6.
92. Richards S, Aziz N, Bale S, et al. Standards and guidelines for the interpretation of sequence variants: a joint consensus recommendation of the American College of Medical Genetics and Genomics and the Association for Molecular Pathology. Genet Med 2015;17(5):405–24.
93. Akimoto C, Volk AE, van Blitterswijk M, et al. A blinded international study on the reliability of genetic testing for GGGGCC-repeat expansions in C9orf72 reveals marked differences in results among 14 laboratories. J Med Genet 2014;51(6): 419–24.
94. Rollinson S, Bennion Callister J, Young K, et al. Small deletion in C9orf72 hides a proportion of expansion carriers in FTLD. Neurobiol Aging 2015;36(3):1601.e1-5.
95. Klepek H, Goutman SA, Quick A, et al. Variable reporting of C9orf72 and a high rate of uncertain results in ALS genetic testing. Neurol Genet 2019;5(1):e301.
96. Gijselinck I, Van Mossevelde S, van der Zee J, et al. The C9orf72 repeat size correlates with onset age of disease, DNA methylation and transcriptional downregulation of the promoter. Mol Psychiatry 2016;21(8):1112–24.

Diagnostic and Prognostic Laboratory Testing for Alzheimer Disease

Zachary Winder, BS[a], Donna Wilcock, PhD[a],
Gregory A. Jicha, MD, PhD[b],*

KEYWORDS

- Alzheimer's disease • Mild cognitive impairment (MCI) • Preclinical AD
- β-amyloid (Aβ) • Tau • Phospho-tau • Cerebrospinal fluid (CSF)

KEY POINTS

- Alzheimer disease is recognized as a slowly progressive continuum, spanning early pre-clinical pathologic change without clinical symptoms to an early state of memory impairment without functional decline, referred to as mild cognitive impairment, to the classically recognized Alzheimer disease stage of dementia.
- The sensitivity and specificity of unique laboratory biomarkers vary across stages of disease that parallel the pathologic processes at play across the Alzheimer continuum.
- Commercially available laboratory biomarkers that are approved by the Food and Drug Administration include cerebrospinal fluid β-amyloid and tau assays as well as genetic testing for autosomal dominant forms of Alzheimer disease and the highly prevalent apolipoprotein E isotype assay.
- Advances in the field include efforts to validate peripheral blood-derived biomarkers as well as to expand the biomarker repertoire to include other markers of neurodegeneration, such as neurofilament light, inflammation, and cell type–specific exosomal markers, among others.

OVERVIEW OF ALZHEIMER DISEASE AND LABORATORY-BASED BIOMARKERS

Alzheimer disease (AD) is the most prevalent of all neurodegenerative disorders, affecting more than 46.8 million persons across the globe today.[1] This number is expected to increase dramatically to more than 131.5 million by the year 2050 with the extension of the life span afforded by modern medical care.[1] AD traditionally has

[a] Department of Physiology, Sanders-Brown Center on Aging, University of Kentucky College of Medicine, 800 South Limestone Street, Lexington, KY 40536-0230, USA; [b] Department of Neurology, Sanders-Brown Center on Aging, University of Kentucky College of Medicine, 800 South Limestone Street, Lexington, KY 40536-0230, USA
* Corresponding author. Sanders-Brown Center on Aging, 1030 South Broadway, Suite #5, Lexington, KY 40504.
E-mail address: gajich2@email.uky.edu

Clin Lab Med 40 (2020) 289–303
https://doi.org/10.1016/j.cll.2020.05.003
0272-2712/20/© 2020 Elsevier Inc. All rights reserved.

labmed.theclinics.com

been recognized clinically only at the stage of dementia, where cognitive decline is severe enough to impact daily function; however, advances in understanding of this disease over the past 2 decades have led to an appreciation that the pathologic processes eventually leading to dementia take decades to occur, progressing through several stages of disease (**Table 1**).[2] This has led to the development of diagnostic criteria for AD, including a prodromal clinical stage, referred to as mild cognitive impairment (MCI), where cognition is impaired but function remains relatively intact and advanced pathology may be present.[2] Research criteria also been have developed for the clinically silent phase of disease, where overt cognitive symptoms essentially are undetectable but pathologic changes, detectable only through the use of laboratory and imaging biomarkers, are present, referred to as preclinical AD (**Fig. 1**).[2] The development and use of biomarkers are essential for accurate diagnostic categorization not only of AD at the dementia stage but more importantly at the prodromal and preclinical stages, where biomarkers actually define the disease beyond clinical signs and symptoms.[2]

Classically, a diagnosis of definite AD could only be made at autopsy, through the demonstration of neuronal degeneration in the presence of both cortical β-amyloid (Aβ) plaques and neurofibrillary degeneration, including both tangles and dystrophic neurites (see **Fig. 1**A and C).[3] The development of diagnostic biomarkers in the field of imaging as well as in laboratory testing has now made a definitive diagnosis of AD possible in a living patient.[2,4] The development of molecular laboratory and imaging biomarkers has increased understanding of the pathologic processes at play in the preclinical AD, prodromal MCI, and dementia stages of disease.[2] Current understanding of these processes suggests that accumulation of amyloid throughout cortical regions, associated with a reduction in cerebrospinal fluid (CSF) Aβ, is followed by synaptic dysfunction engendered by the influences of soluble oligomeric Aβ species, neuronal injury, and the advent of abnormal post-translational changes in the microtubule-associated protein tau, leading to disruption of the neuronal cytoskeleton in the development of intraneuronal neurofibrillary tangles (see **Table 1**).[2] As these processes progress, markers of oxidative stress, glial activation and resultant inflammation, and neuronal death signal progression of disease.[2,5,6] These factors also may play early roles in the development of pathology and much ongoing research is exploring such mechanisms as either causative or contributory to the disease process.

Given scientific advances in the understanding of the pathophysiology of AD, multiple new classes of potentially disease-modifying therapies are being brought to bear in early clinical testing as a cure for this devastating disease is searched for.[7] The currently approved and available therapies for AD are nonspecific to disease processes and primary pathologic diagnosis.[7] As such, the need for definitive

Table 1
Spectrum of Alzheimer disease from prebiological through dementia stages

Characteristic	Prebiological Stage	Preclinical Stage	Prodromal Stage (Mild Cognitive Impairment)	Dementia Stage
Genetic risk	+/−	+/−	+/−	+/−
Aβ accumulation	−	+	+	+
Tau abnormalities	−	+/−	+	+
Neurodegeneration	−	+/−	+	+
Cognitive decline	−	−	+	+
Functional decline	−	−	−	+

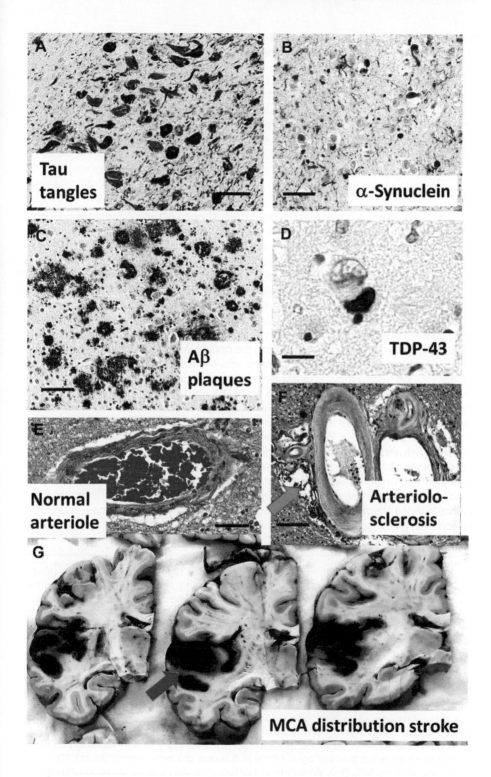

biomarker-based diagnosis for the disease remains largely academic. This is expected to change dramatically once disease and molecular mechanism–specific therapies are proved and implemented in the course of standard clinical care.[2,5,6] At present, laboratory-based biomarkers for AD all rest on the collection of CSF.[4–6,8] Ideally, blood-based biomarkers would facilitate widespread use of such testing; however, the sensitivity and specificity of such peripheral laboratory testing remain challenging for the field.[6,9–14] The need for low-cost, noninvasive biomarkers will be critical for treatment selection in the future, once specific disease-modifying therapies are brought into routine clinical use.[7]

THE GENETICS OF ALZHEIMER DISEASE

Advances in understanding of the genetic contributions to AD also have led to concomitant advances in the development of laboratory testing to identify genetic predisposition and risk for the subsequent development of the disease.[15] Several mutations in 3 specific genes are causative of autosomal dominant AD.[15] Persons with such mutations tend to experience the onset of clinical AD in their fifth or sixth decade of life, and approximately 50% of each successive generation is affected, consistent with the autosomal dominant nature of these mutations.[15] Commercially available, Food and Drug Administration (FDA)-approved testing for mutations in the amyloid precursor protein (APP) gene on chromosome 21, presenilin 1 (PS1) gene on chromosome 14, and presenilin 2 (PS2) gene on chromosome 1 affords the opportunity to test for such forms of disease long before the pathologic processes and/or clinical manifestations of disease appear.[15] Such testing may be useful for reproductive planning as well as future prognosis and can be used to identify individuals at risk for disease to facilitate primary and secondary prevention studies using novel therapeutics. Such mutations, however, are quite rare and lead to less than 1% of the prevalence of AD cases globally.[15]

For almost 2.5 decades, it has been understood that genes that may modify and increase AD risk are prevalent in the population. Such mutations are incompletely penetrant and do not absolutely determine the future presence and/or absence of AD. The first such gene identified in this category codes for the apolipoprotein E, epsilon 4 (ε4) allele.[15,16] Such mutations are relatively common in the population, are seen with increasing frequency in those affected by AD, and increase risk of disease in a gene-dose–dependent fashion, with homozygotes at greatest risk.[15,16] Commercially available, FDA-approved

---

Fig. 1. Representative pathologies in a 93-year-old woman followed to death with a clinical dementia rating score = 0 (normal cognition), highlighting pathologic features that often are mixed in the same individual and that may be present even during the presymptomatic phase of disease. AD neurofibrillary tangles, comprised largely of abnormal tau protein in the amygdala visualized by PHF-1 immunohistochemistry (original magnification ×20) (A); intraneuronal Lewy bodies and Lewy neurites visualized with α-synuclein immunohistochemistry (original magnification ×10) in the amygdala (B); extracellular Aβ plaques characteristic of AD in the amygdala visualized by Aβ immunohistochemistry (original magnification ×10) (C); TDP-43 intraneuronal inclusions in the amygdala visualized by immunohistochemistry (original magnification ×60) (D); pathologic sections demonstrating a normal arteriole (E [hematoxylin-eosin stain, original magnification ×4]) and arteriolosclerosis (F [hematoxylin-eosin stain, original magnification ×4]); gross photographs of a large parietal middle cerebral artery (MCA) infarction (G). Arrow in F is expanded Virchow Robin space with inflammation. At higher power, these inflammatory cells included lymphocytes and hemosiderin-laden macrophages. Arrow in G shows the hemorrhagic infarct. (*Courtesy of* Dr. Peter Nelson, MD, PhD, University of Kentucky Sanders-Brown Center on Aging.)

testing for ε4 allele expression frequently is used in clinical practice, although the current position statement by the American Academy of Neurology discourages such testing, given a limited ability to use this knowledge in a clinically meaningful way.[17] Yet, much evidence is accumulating that the efficacy and safety of both currently approved and experimental therapies may be influenced by this genetic risk factor. It is possible in the near future that routine testing for the ε4 allele may become part of standard clinical practice.[16] Since this initial discovery, facilitated by technological developments in genetic research, more than a dozen other genes influencing risk for AD have been identified (**Table 2**).[15] These genes are linked to several common pathways, including cholesterol trafficking, inflammation, synaptic function, and even brain development.[15] Not only are such discoveries being developed into new genetic tests, many of which are focusing on polygenic risk scores for disease, but also they are identifying new targets for disease-modifying therapeutic intervention.[18,19]

PATHOLOGIC HETEROGENEITY AND THE CONUNDRUM OF MIXED DEMENTIA

Although the promise of an improved repertoire of low-cost, noninvasive disease-specific biomarkers for AD looms on the near horizon, the field remains questionably skeptical regarding the practical use of such biomarkers given an emerging under-standing of the inherent pathologic heterogeneity seen in most cases of late-onset AD (see **Fig. 1**).[2,5,8,20] Although autosomal dominant AD affecting a younger popula-tion typically can present as a pathologically pure entity, virtually every community-based autopsy cohort of typical late-onset AD has demonstrated that mixed pathology is the rule rather than the exception.[3,20] Common comorbid pathologic features seen in AD at autopsy include cerebrovascular disease (CVD), Lewy body pathology (LBP) characterized by α-synuclein inclusions, and the more recently described TAR DNA-binding protein 43 (TDP-43) inclusions (see **Fig. 1**, which demonstrates that all com-mon comorbid pathologic features of a mixed dementia state can be seen in the same individual, even when the disease remains clinically silent).[3,20] Defining AD using antemortem laboratory biomarkers will remain limited in utility until such time as bio-markers for these common comorbid pathologic states are developed.

CVD increases with age similar to AD, leading to a common overlap in pathologic features, especially in those with advanced age. In most cases, CVD contributions to cognitive and functional decline include insidious, slowly progressive, small vessel ischemic change rather than overt small or large vessel stroke presenting with acute and/or stepwise decline (see **Fig. 1**). This creates a clinical confound in diagnosis un-less imaging is used to identify the cerebrovascular injury. In addition, many of the most common CVD risk factors also are widely recognized as common risk factors for AD. Although magnetic resonance imaging is considered the hallmark biomarker for CVD, large-scale efforts are under way to develop laboratory testing for dementia caused by CVD that may exist independently or frequently in conjunction with AD.[21] The MarkVCID consortium efforts, currently funded by the National Institute of Neuro-logical Disorders and Stroke, is leading such efforts in the United States, and several blood-based and CSF-based biomarkers have been proposed for exploration that may well lead to the future development of laboratory testing for this common comor-bid pathology in AD.

Although LBP is characteristic of Parkinson disease and dementia with Lewy bodies (DLB) in its pure form, it can be seen commonly as a comorbid pathology in up to 50% of autopsy confirmed cases of AD (see **Fig. 1**B).[20] Frequently such cases do not meet criteria for either Parkinson disease or DLB, so the development of antemortem laboratory-based biomarkers for α-synuclein pathology is critical for accurate

Table 2
Genetic risks for Alzheimer disease

Gene	Mechanism	Population Prevalence (%)	Disease Risk Conferred (%)	Commercial Testing Available
APP	Autosomal dominant, chromosomal triplication (Down syndrome), autosomal recessive	<1	100	Yes
Presenilin 1 (PSEN1)	Autosomal dominant	<1	100	Yes
Presenilin 2 (PSEN2)	Autosomal dominant	<1	100	Yes
Apolipoprotein E (ε4 allele)	Allelic variation, cholesterol trafficking, increases Aβ	14%	30–75	Yes
Clusterin/apolipoprotein J (CLU)	Cholesterol trafficking/synapse function	38	14	No
ABCA7	Lipid metabolism	19	15	No
SORL1	Lipid metabolism	4	23	No
CD2AP	Endocytosis/cytoskeletal organization	27	10	No
PICALM	Synapse function	36	13	No
BIN1	Synapse function	41	22	No
CR1	Immune function	20	18	No
CD33	Immune function	31	6	No
MS4A	Immune function	40	10	No
TREM2	Immune function	<1	35	No
EPHA1	Brain development	34	10	No

This list contains the major genetic risk variants identified to date but is not all-inclusive. Increasing allelic frequency in the general population appears to be associated with lesser risk for AD. The genes appear to be related to functional pathways involved in amyloid generation, lipid metabolism and trafficking, synapse function and endocytosis, immune function and inflammatory pathways, and brain development.

diagnostic testing of AD, when mixed pathology may play a critical role in prognosis and/or optimal selection of therapeutic interventions.[20] Previous work has demonstrated that the coexistence of AD and LBP lead to a more aggressive phenotype of disease that has wide-reaching implications for both prognosis and clinical care. Currently approved laboratory and/or imaging biomarkers for LBP in Parkinson disease or DLB are lacking in the diagnostic repertoire, yet much promising research is under way. It is hoped that such biomarkers will become available in the near future that may help sort out the question of whether or not LBP is associated with the AD pathology that already can be diagnosed with laboratory biomarkers as responsible for the dementia seen clinically.

TDP-43 was identified in 2006 is a major protein constituent of the ubiquitin-aided inclusions characteristic of frontotemporal dementia and amyotrophic lateral sclerosis.[20,22] The original publications following this discovery highlighted the frequent comorbidity of AD and TDP-43 pathology in autopsy cases of clinically diagnosed AD.[22] Since that time, multiple community-based autopsy cohorts of late-onset AD have described the coexistence of TDP-43 pathology with AD pathology in up to 50% of cases (see **Fig. 1**D).[20,22] It also has been noted that TDP-43 pathology, frequently associated with age-related hippocampal sclerosis, is a common clinical mimic of AD.[23] The importance of these findings is underscored by a recent consensus statement from an international working group assembled by the National Institute on Aging, that named this unique pathology, limbic-associated TDP-43 encephalopathy (LATE).[23] As such, antemortem laboratory and/or imaging-based biomarkers of TDP-43 pathology have become an important focus of laboratory-based biomarker research. The ability to identify TDP-43 pathology is responsible for the clinical syndrome of AD and/or as a comorbid pathologic feature of AD is critically important, as with LBP, both for prognosis and for optimal therapeutic interventional selection for persons with clinical AD diagnoses.[20,23]

Several other pathologic entities that involve tau inclusions, such as primary age-related tauopathy, argyrophilic grain disease, progressive supranuclear palsy (PSP), cortical-basal degeneration (CBD), and aging-related tau astrogliopathy also are confounding to laboratory testing for AD in regard to both diagnosis and prognosis.[24] Given that extant AD laboratory biomarkers focus at least partially on the detection of tau pathology, such comorbid pathology could introduce bias in the interpretation of laboratory-based AD biomarkers. In addition, current methodologies utilized in commercially available, FDA-approved assays largely are unable to distinguish tau isoform expression profiles and/or post-translational modifications that may distinguish these diseases that appear to have convergent neurodegenerative mechanisms involving tau protein. Fortunately for the field, comorbid tau-related, nontangle/neurite pathology in AD is less common than that seen with CVD, LBD, and TDP-43 pathology. Nonetheless, further work refining the ability to diagnose-specific pathologic disease states in which tau serves as a biomarker is critical for advancement in the field.

COMMERCIALLY AVAILABLE CEREBROSPINAL TESTING FOR ALZHEIMER DISEASE

CSF testing for Aβ and tau protein has been available for many years as an FDA-approved test for AD.[6,8,25] Although this test does rely on an invasive procedure, spinal tap or lumbar puncture as it is commonly referred to, it appears highly accurate in determining pathology for the 2 hallmark pathologies of AD, amyloid plaques and neurofibrillary tangles.[6,8,25] This test is used as frequently to rule out AD as it is to rule in the pathology and as such its primary utility is in those subjects for whom the question of underlying diagnosis remains unclear. The test itself is available for approximately $1000 and frequently is covered by insurance. The ordering physician may need to justify the need for this test in order to obtain third-party coverage. Both the invasiveness of the CSF collection procedure and the potential for noncoverage have limited the widespread use of CSF testing to confirm the diagnosis of AD in many clinics. The test itself typically focuses on measurement of the Aβ 1-42 fragment, total tau levels, and the detection of levels of tau phosphorylated at specific residues. Understanding each of these components is critical for accurate interpretation of the diagnostic testing performed.

The APP is a common membrane-bound glycoprotein subserving normal cellular functions, including neuronal plasticity and response to acute injury among others, that typically is cleaved by both an alpha secretase and beta secretase to yield a readily clearable amyloid fragment.[26] In AD, the cleavage typically entails a beta secretase and gamma secretase–generated fragment that can vary in the number of amino acid residues but typically is found as either a 42 or 40 amino acid fragment.[26] Although alpha secretase and beta secretase cleave APP in its extracellular domain, gamma secretase cleaves this membrane-bound protein within the hydrophobic intramembrane domain, producing a fragment that is highly prone to aggregate within the highly charged extracellular CSF.[26] Aβ fragments first form soluble oligomeric complexes, which have been shown to be highly synaptotoxic, interfering with long-term potentiation and memory formation as well as leading to direct cellular injury.[26] Eventually aggregation leads to the formation of insoluble filaments, which begin to accumulate within the extracellular brain parenchyma to form the characteristic dense core and neuritic plaques of AD.[26] Although both the 42 and 40 amino acid forms are found within parenchymal amyloid plaques, the 40 amino acid form has a predilection for accumulation within the cerebral microvasculature, including small arterials in capillaries.[26] Such accumulation leads to cerebral amyloid angiopathy, which can predispose to vascular injury, including both microhemorrhage and macrohemorrhage. Commercially available assays focus on measurement of the 42 amino acid form.

Tau is one of many intracellular microtubule-associated proteins that normally serves to stabilize the alpha and beta tubulin arrays responsible for the stable neuronal cytoskeleton.[27] Upon phosphorylation of certain residues, tau dissociates from the microtubule array, destabilizing it and leading to dissolution of the neuronal cytoskeleton.[27] Under normal conditions, this process allows remodeling of the neuronal cytoskeleton to form new connections and allow learning and memory to occur. In AD, tau is hyperphosphorylated and undergoes conformational change, creating a beta pleated sheet conformation that is highly prone to aggregation of tau and the eventual formation of paired helical filaments, which in turn aggregate to form the neurofibrillary tangles and dystrophic neurites of AD.[27] Both phosphorylation-independent and phosphorylation-dependent epitopes are included in the commercially available AD laboratory tests. Phosphorylation-independent levels of tau correlate highly with degree of neuronal cell death but do not include disease-specific phosphorylation event detection.[8,25,27] Specific phosphorylations are thought to be relatively disease specific, so the use of phospho-tau epitope detection increases the specificity for the AD disease state.[27] The choice of specific tau phospho-epitope potentially could dramatically affect the specificity and sensitivity of the test.[8,27] In addition, tau isoform expression can be unique in unique disease states.[27] Although AD classically involves aggregates composed of all isoforms, specific forms of frontotemporal dementia or caused by tau mutations that lead to overexpression of either a 3 or 4 repeat tau isoform.[27] Three repeat tau inclusions are characteristic of Pick disease, a form of frontotemporal dementia, whereas 4 repeat inclusions can be characteristic of frontotemporal dementia related to tau mutations, PSP, and CBD.[27] The development of commercially available tests recognizing differential isoform expression and or conformational changes in tau remain elusive but could add specificity for tau-related comorbidities and/or disease states as well as enhance the specificity and sensitivity for AD pathology.

Commercially available, FDA-approved CSF testing typically includes both analysis of amyloid-to-tau ratio and assessment of phosphorylated tau (p-tau) levels. In AD CSF, free Aβ is reduced as it is being deposited preferentially in the parenchyma, whereas cell death is increasing total tau protein levels.[8,26] Utilizing these 2 measures in a ratio increases sensitivity for detecting and AD state. The addition of an assay for p-tau increases the specificity for in AD state. P-tau levels should increase with increasing AD pathophysiology. Absolute levels of Aβ 1-42, total tau, and phospho-tau, however, can be quite variable in the aging population irrespective of the presence or absence of AD pathology.[8,26] As such, the use of the specific measures cross-sectionally in a unique individual requires this combination rather than a single test for absolute determination of AD status. Increased understanding of the longitudinal course of these biomarkers has suggested that within-subject change actually may be much more predictive than absolute levels.[8,26] The same holds true, albeit at a magnified extent, for AD assays in serum or plasma. Both sensitivity and specificity of such tests suggest that their primary use is in tracking the longitudinal progression of an individual rather than differentiating individuals in diagnosing disease at a single point in time.[5,6,8,9,12,14,28] Technological developments improving the accuracy of such assays and/or beginning to consider isolating subfractions and/or exosomal fractions of these proteins may help overcome the barriers inherent in the development of noninvasive blood-based biomarkers for AD.[29,30]

ISSUES INHERENT IN COMMERCIALLY AVAILABLE TESTING FOR GENETIC PREDISPOSITION TO ALZHEIMER DISEASE

Given the rarity of autosomal dominant forms of AD as well as the under-appreciation of the incomplete penetrance of Alzheimer risk genes that vary in regard to both penetrance and degree of influence on subsequent development of Alzheimer pathology, genetic testing for AD is not part of the routine clinical experience in most settings.[15] Issues specific for the understanding and interpretation of both autosomal dominant and genetic risk testing need to be incorporated into routine clinical practice before such tests begin to be collected for the purposes of general diagnostic and/or prognostic determination.[16] Such issues have been addressed in the setting of research studies that have included disclosure to individuals but have yet to be adapted for routine clinical practice.

Testing for autosomal dominant mutation should be restricted to patients with a family pedigree and clinical presentation for affected relatives consistent with understanding of the autosomal dominant forms of AD.[17] This should include familial pedigrees, demonstrating approximately 50% of individuals affected in each subsequent generation as well as the earlier age of onset for affected individuals. Routine genetic testing for autosomal dominant mutations in AD should not be performed if the familial pedigree does not suggest an autosomal dominant form of transmission and or in instances where the age of onset is in the sixth or greater decade of life. Considerations for why autosomal dominant genetic testing would be pursued follow the recommendations for other autosomal dominant inherited neurologic diseases, such as future reproductive planning, and/or later life planning for management of individual resources, and/or care needs and respect for advanced care planning, such as advance directives and living will considerations. Formal genetic counseling consultation is recommended before pursuing testing for autosomal dominant AD, as with other inherited disorders.

Genetic testing for risk genes, such as the ε4 allele of the apolipoprotein E gene, while routinely done for research purposes, currently is not recommended by the American Academy of Neurology because it has little bearing on diagnosis, prognosis, or treatment decisions.[17] Several research studies have disclosed ε4 allele status and have found that disclosure of such results in increased anxiety and apprehension regarding the possibility of impending AD but otherwise appears to have no negative influences on quality of life and/or lifestyle decisions.[31,32] A general lack of education of both the general population as well as health care professionals that might seek out such testing, however, limits the ability of such testing to truly inform decisions, such as those under consideration for individuals and families potentially at risk for autosomal dominant AD. The situation may well change in the future. Previous data, including a clinical trial in MCI, demonstrated that the potential benefit of treatment with currently available medications (donepezil) may be more beneficial for those who are ε4 allele carriers than in those who lack the ε4 allele.[33] Studies of experimental medicines using active and passive immunization against Aβ demonstrate increased risk for side effects, which can be devastating, including cerebral edema, stroke, and hemorrhage.[34] As such, ε4 allele testing has become routine in such studies, potentially paving the way for FDA approval of such medications depending on prior ε4 allele testing. But for now, avoiding such genetic testing is in the benefit of patients and should not be pursued unless extenuating circumstances are present and appropriate genetic counseling is pursued.[17]

ADDITIONAL EXPERIMENTAL BIOMARKERS CURRENTLY UNDER EVALUATION
Plasma Alzheimer Disease Biomarkers

As previously outlined, both Aβ and tau can be quantified in CSF samples in order to assist in the diagnosis of AD. CSF draws, however, are both invasive and expensive to perform on all individuals at risk of developing AD. Blood draws, on the other hand, are performed regularly during routine clinical evaluations and, therefore, are an attractive method to obtain potential fluid biomarkers for AD.[9,12] Efforts have been undertaken to evaluate Aβ and tau levels in blood plasma to understand the relationship with their CSF counterpart in addition to differentiating patients with AD from appropriate controls.[14] Although plasma $Aβ_{42}$ appears to have mixed results for significant correlations with CSF $Aβ_{42}$, the ratio of $Aβ_{42}/Aβ_{40}$ does show more consistency in having a significant relationship between plasma and CSF findings.[13,35–37] These results show that plasma quantification of these proteins may provide similar information to that which can be obtained from CSF measurements. The ratio of $Aβ_{42}/Aβ_{40}$ also has been shown to differentiate patients with AD from cognitively normal and non-AD dementia controls, with AD patients with having a significantly lower ratio of $Aβ_{42}/Aβ_{40}$ compared with controls across multiple cohorts of patients.[13,35,36] This generalizability through multiple studies provides evidence for the use of such a ratio as an alternative to the current commercially available CSF biomarkers.

Plasma levels of p-tau-181 also have been shown significantly increased in patients with AD compared with controls and significantly correlated with levels in the CSF.[28] Such use provides another alternative to the more invasive and expensive CSF protein quantifications at play presently. Studies to determine whether plasma $Aβ_{42}$ and $Aβ_{40}$ could differentiate preclinical forms of AD were shown to be unsuccessful.[10] This finding highlights the important limitation of many biomarkers for AD, which may vary in results depending on the disease stage. Despite such limitations, plasma quantifications of $A\beta_{42}$, $A\beta_{40}$, and p-tau offer a potential alternative to the FDA-approved CSF quantifications of these proteins for differentiating patients with AD from cognitively normal individuals. A continued need to develop biomarkers that can monitor the progression of disease may require additional fluid biomarkers that might preferentially characterize discrete stages in the disease process.

Inflammatory Biomarkers

Activated microglia are prominent pathologic findings in patients with AD.[38] These microglia stimulate an inflammatory phenotype throughout the brain, which has been characterized in the CSF and plasma.[6] Unlike traditional biomarkers associated with AD, some inflammatory biomarkers have been shown to differentiate patients at different stages of AD and can serve to monitor the progression of the disease. These markers are interesting for their ability to track disease progression but remain in a preliminary stage of study.

Biomarkers of interest include CSF levels of visinin-like protein-1 (VILIP-1) and chitinase-3-like protein 1 (YKL-40). VILIP-1 previously has been identified as a neuronal marker up-regulated in stroke-related injuries and YKL-40 is a protein implicated in neuroinflammation. YKL-40 was shown to differentiate MCI and AD patients from cognitively normal controls[39,40] and interestingly was significantly elevated in patients with MCI who progressed to AD on follow-up, average 2.7 years later. Similar elevations of VILIP-1 in patients progressing to AD also were seen.[39]

Another biomarker that has been shown significantly elevated across multiple studies of CSF samples in MCI and AD patients compared with controls is soluble triggering receptor expressed on myeloid cells 2 (sTREM2).[6] Mutations in TREM2 have been shown to have increased risk of developing AD,[41] so it is not surprising that changes in sTREM2 correlate to the clinical diagnosis of AD. Multiple studies have found the highest CSF levels of sTREM2 during the MCI phase of the disease, indicating a potential peak prior to the development of AD. Plasma levels of sTREM2, however, were not able to differentiate AD from control patients, which may lessen the feasibility of this biomarker for clinical use as the field turns toward development of blood based biomarkers as a central focus of exploration.[42,43]

A recent meta-analysis provides insights into additional inflammatory biomarkers, which previously may have been overlooked. In particular, 51 peripherally measured analytes evaluated through 175 studies have been identified, with 19 being significantly different in patients with AD and controls, but larger clinical trials still are needed to demonstrate the generalizability of these biomarkers.[44]

Exosomal Biomarkers

Exosomes are small vesicles secreted from cells, which can be used to remove proteins and communicate with other cells.[29] Exosomes can identify cell lineage or source via cell-surface markers.[29] Cell-specific exosomes then can be used to characterize pathologic processes occurring in the specific cell types from which they were produced.[29] This additional information provides key insights into cellular processes occurring in various disease states and makes them unique as cell type–specific biomarkers. Two exosomal cell types that have piqued interest in the field include astrocyte-derived exosomes (ADEs) and neuronal-derived exosomes (NDEs). Differences between patients with AD and controls suggest that such cell-specific samples may allow development of biomarkers for diagnosis as well as providing a foundation to begin to understand the mechanistic interplay between astrocytes and neurons throughout different stages of AD.[30,45]

Plasma ADEs, when compared between patients with AD and cognitively normal controls, showed significantly higher levels of inflammatory markers (interleukin [IL]-6, tumor necrosis factor α, and IL-1β), increased levels of complement effector proteins, and decreased levels of complement regulatory proteins.[30] Two of those complement regulatory proteins, CD59 and DAF, also were shown to be decreased in individuals with preclinical AD and decreased further in patients diagnosed with AD.[30] Plasma NDEs also have been shown to have decreased presynaptic proteins and postsynaptic receptors, which are hypothesized to be indicative of neuronal damage in AD.[45] Four proteins were evaluated, AMP4A, NPTX2, NLGN1, and NRXN2, where all were significantly decreased in AD patients compared with controls. Additionally, all but NPTX2 were decreased in preclinical AD, with a further decrease in diagnosed AD patients.[45] Although these results are promising and use easily accessible plasma samples, exosome evaluation is still a relatively new technique and will be required to be conducted in larger studies before generalizability and feasibility for widespread use can be determined.

Neurofilament Light

Neurofilament light (NFL) is a component of the neurofilament protein, which is found in the axonal cytoskeleton.[46] When neurons are damaged, as in AD, neurofilament is released into the blood and CSF, where it can be quantified and used as a biomarker for evaluating neuronal damage.[46] Studies have been conducted measuring NFL in plasma, serum, and CSF, where NFL levels appeared to be correlated for plasma and CSF[11] as well as serum and CSF.[11,47] Plasma NFL levels were shown significantly elevated not only in AD compared with controls but also in patients with MCI compared with controls and in AD compared with MCI.[11,46,48] Serum NFL also has shown effectiveness as a biomarker in evaluating conversion of asymptomatic AD in autosomal dominant mutation carriers to symptomatic AD based on the rate of serum NFL change. Converters from asymptomatic to symptomatic AD had increased serum NFL change compared with those who remained asymptomatic from baseline to follow-up testing.[49] These studies provide evidence for the continued testing of an NFL biomarker to both evaluate and monitor disease progression in individuals at risk of developing AD in both the presymptomatic and MCI phases of the disease. NFL, however, is a nonspecific biomarker of accelerated neuronal death and degeneration, so may lack specificity for the AD disease state despite the strong data supporting its use in tracking disease progression.

SUMMARY

The increasing prevalence of AD worldwide has necessitated more efficient methods for diagnosis and potential treatment of individuals affected by the disease. The necessity for biomarker development to achieve this goal is further propelled by recognition of a multidecade course of disease progression in which recognition of the disease at preclinical stages is of paramount importance. The current state of laboratory assays as biomarkers for AD diagnosis is limited to Aβ and tau analysis of CSF samples. Discoveries in the field, however, are rapidly evolving, moving forward the exploration of blood-based biomarkers for ease of sampling procedures and the exploration of a host of disease-associated features, including inflammatory biomarkers and cell-specific exosomal biomarkers that may help diagnose AD more accurately as well as track disease progression in AD. The field anticipates new commercially available assays that are FDA approved for such clinical use in the near future.

DISCLOSURE

Dr G.A. Jicha has provided contract research services for AbbVie. Alltech, Biohaven, Eisai, Janssen, Lilly, Novartis, and Suven. The other authors have nothing to disclose.

REFERENCES

1. Patterson C, Lynch C, Bliss A, et al. World Alzheimer Report 2018. Alzheimer Disease International (ADI). London, UK. Available at: https://www.alz.co.uk/research/world-report-2018.
2. Jack CR Jr, Bennett DA, Blennow K, et al. NIA-AA research framework: toward a biological definition of Alzheimer's disease. Alzheimers Dement 2018;14(4): 535–62.
3. Montine TJ, Monsell SE, Beach TG, et al. Multisite assessment of NIA-AA guidelines for the neuropathologic evaluation of Alzheimer's disease. Alzheimers Dement 2016;12(2):164–9.
4. Dubois B, Hampel H, Feldman HH, et al. Preclinical Alzheimer's disease: definition, natural history, and diagnostic criteria. Alzheimers Dement 2016;12(3): 292–323.
5. Guzman-Martinez L, Maccioni RB, Farias GA, et al. Biomarkers for Alzheimer's disease. Curr Alzheimer Res 2019;16(6):518–28.
6. Lashley T, Schott JM, Weston P, et al. Molecular biomarkers of Alzheimer's disease: progress and prospects. Dis Model Mech 2018;11(5) [pii:dmm031781].
7. Cummings J, Aisen PS, DuBois B, et al. Drug development in Alzheimer's disease: the path to 2025. Alzheimers Res Ther 2016;8:39.
8. Lewczuk P, Riederer P, O'Bryant SE, et al. Cerebrospinal fluid and blood biomarkers for neurodegenerative dementias: an update of the consensus of the task force on biological markers in psychiatry of the World Federation of Societies of biological Psychiatry. World J Biol Psychiatry 2018;19(4):244–328.
9. Hampel H, O'Bryant SE, Molinuevo JL, et al. Blood-based biomarkers for Alzheimer disease: mapping the road to the clinic. Nat Rev Neurol 2018;14(11): 639–52.
10. Lovheim H, Elgh F, Johansson A, et al. Plasma concentrations of free amyloid beta cannot predict the development of Alzheimer's disease. Alzheimers Dement 2017;13(7):778–82.
11. Mattsson N, Andreasson U, Zetterberg H, et al. Association of plasma neurofilament light with neurodegeneration in patients with Alzheimer disease. JAMA Neurol 2017;74(5):557–66.
12. O'Bryant SE, Mielke MM, Rissman RA, et al. Blood-based biomarkers in Alzheimer disease: current state of the science and a novel collaborative paradigm for advancing from discovery to clinic. Alzheimers Dement 2017;13(1):45–58.
13. Vogelgsang J, Shahpasand-Kroner H, Vogelgsang R, et al. Multiplex immunoassay measurement of amyloid-beta42 to amyloid-beta40 ratio in plasma discriminates between dementia due to Alzheimer's disease and dementia not due to Alzheimer's disease. Exp Brain Res 2018;236(5):1241–50.
14. Zetterberg H, Burnham SC. Blood-based molecular biomarkers for Alzheimer's disease. Mol Brain 2019;12(1):26.
15. Chouraki V, Seshadri S. Genetics of Alzheimer's disease. Adv Genet 2014;87: 245–94.
16. Seshadri S, Drachman DA, Lippa CF. Apolipoprotein E epsilon 4 allele and the lifetime risk of Alzheimer's disease. What physicians know, and what they should know. Arch Neurol 1995;52(11):1074–9.

17. Knopman DS, DeKosky ST, Cummings JL, et al. Practice parameter: diagnosis of dementia (an evidence-based review). Report of the quality standards Subcommittee of the American Academy of Neurology. Neurology 2001;56(9):1143–53.

18. Escott-Price V, Shoai M, Pither R, et al. Polygenic score prediction captures nearly all common genetic risk for Alzheimer's disease. Neurobiol Aging 2017; 49:214.e7-11.

19. Tan CH, Bonham LW, Fan CC, et al. Polygenic hazard score, amyloid deposition and Alzheimer's neurodegeneration. Brain 2019;142(2):460–70.

20. Boyle PA, Yu L, Wilson RS, et al. Person-specific contribution of neuropathologies to cognitive loss in old age. Ann Neurol 2018;83(1):74–83.

21. Cipollini V, Troili F, Giubilei F. Emerging biomarkers in vascular cognitive impairment and dementia: from pathophysiological pathways to clinical application. Int J Mol Sci 2019;20(11) [pii:E2812].

22. Chen-Plotkin AS, Lee VM, Trojanowski JQ. TAR DNA-binding protein 43 in neurodegenerative disease. Nat Rev Neurol 2010;6(4):211–20.

23. Nelson PT, Dickson DW, Trojanowski JQ, et al. Limbic-predominant age-related TDP-43 encephalopathy (LATE): consensus working group report. Brain 2019; 142(6):1503–27.

24. Jicha GA, Nelson PT. Hippocampal sclerosis, argyrophilic grain disease, and primary age-related tauopathy. Continuum (Minneap Minn) 2019;25(1):208–33.

25. Alexopoulos P, Roesler J, Thierjung N, et al. Mapping CSF biomarker profiles onto NIA-AA guidelines for Alzheimer's disease. Eur Arch Psychiatry Clin Neurosci 2016;266(7):587–97.

26. Chen XQ, Mobley WC. Alzheimer disease pathogenesis: insights from molecular and cellular biology studies of oligomeric abeta and tau species. Front Neurosci 2019;13:659.

27. Gotz J, Halliday G, Nisbet RM. Molecular pathogenesis of the tauopathies. Annu Rev Pathol 2019;14:239–61.

28. Tatebe H, Kasai T, Ohmichi T, et al. Quantification of plasma phosphorylated tau to use as a biomarker for brain Alzheimer pathology: pilot case-control studies including patients with Alzheimer's disease and down syndrome. Mol Neurodegener 2017;12(1):63.

29. Coleman BM, Hill AF. Extracellular vesicles–Their role in the packaging and spread of misfolded proteins associated with neurodegenerative diseases. Semin Cell Dev Biol 2015;40:89–96.

30. Goetzl EJ, Schwartz JB, Abner EL, et al. High complement levels in astrocyte-derived exosomes of Alzheimer disease. Ann Neurol 2018;83(3):544–52.

31. Chao S, Roberts JS, Marteau TM, et al. Health behavior changes after genetic risk assessment for Alzheimer disease: the REVEAL study. Alzheimer Dis Assoc Disord 2008;22(1):94–7.

32. Guan Y, Roter DL, Erby LH, et al. Disclosing genetic risk of Alzheimer's disease to cognitively impaired patients and visit companions: findings from the REVEAL Study. Patient Educ Couns 2017;100(5):927–35.

33. Petersen RC, Thomas RG, Grundman M, et al. Vitamin E and donepezil for the treatment of mild cognitive impairment. N Engl J Med 2005;352(23):2379–88.

34. Sperling RA, Jack CR Jr, Black SE, et al. Amyloid-related imaging abnormalities in amyloid-modifying therapeutic trials: recommendations from the Alzheimer's Association Research Roundtable Workgroup. Alzheimers Dement 2011;7(4): 367–85.

35. Kim HJ, Park KW, Kim TE, et al. Elevation of the plasma Abeta40/Abeta42 ratio as a diagnostic marker of sporadic early-onset Alzheimer's disease. J Alzheimers Dis 2015;48(4):1043–50.
36. Shahpasand-Kroner H, Klafki HW, Bauer C, et al. A two-step immunoassay for the simultaneous assessment of Abeta38, Abeta40 and Abeta42 in human blood plasma supports the Abeta42/Abeta40 ratio as a promising biomarker candidate of Alzheimer's disease. Alzheimers Res Ther 2018;10(1):121.
37. Verberk IMW, Slot RE, Verfaillie SCJ, et al. Plasma Amyloid as prescreener for the earliest Alzheimer pathological changes. Ann Neurol 2018;84(5):648–58.
38. Glass CK, Saijo K, Winner B, et al. Mechanisms underlying inflammation in neurode-generation. Cell 2010;140(6):918–34.
39. Kester MI, Teunissen CE, Sutphen C, et al. Cerebrospinal fluid VILIP-1 and YKL-40, candidate biomarkers to diagnose, predict and monitor Alzheimer's disease in a memory clinic cohort. Alzheimers Res Ther 2015;7(1):59.
40. Muszynski P, Groblewska M, Kulczynska-Przybik A, et al. YKL-40 as a potential biomarker and a possible target in therapeutic strategies of Alzheimer's disease. Curr Neuropharmacol 2017;15(6):906–17.
41. Guerreiro R, Wojtas A, Bras J, et al. TREM2 variants in Alzheimer's disease. N Engl J Med 2013;368(2):117–27.
42. Liu D, Cao B, Zhao Y, et al. Soluble TREM2 changes during the clinical course of Alzheimer's disease: a meta-analysis. Neurosci Lett 2018;686:10–6.
43. Suarez-Calvet M, Kleinberger G, Araque Caballero MA, et al. sTREM2 cerebro-spinal fluid levels are a potential biomarker for microglia activity in early-stage Alzheimer's disease and associate with neuronal injury markers. EMBO Mol Med 2016;8(5):466–76.
44. Lai KSP, Liu CS, Rau A, et al. Peripheral inflammatory markers in Alzheimer's disease: a systematic review and meta-analysis of 175 studies. J Neurol Neurosurg Psychiatry 2017;88(10):876–82.
45. Goetzl EJ, Abner EL, Jicha GA, et al. Declining levels of functionally specialized synaptic proteins in plasma neuronal exosomes with progression of Alzheimer's disease. FASEB J 2018;32(2):888–93.
46. Lewczuk P, Ermann N, Andreasson U, et al. Plasma neurofilament light as a potential biomarker of neurodegeneration in Alzheimer's disease. Alzheimers Res Ther 2018;10(1):71.
47. Sanchez-Valle R, Heslegrave A, Foiani MS, et al. Serum neurofilament light levels correlate with severity measures and neurodegeneration markers in autosomal dominant Alzheimer's disease. Alzheimers Res Ther 2018;10(1):113.
48. Zhou W, Zhang J, Ye F, et al. Plasma neurofilament light chain levels in Alzheimer's disease. Neurosci Lett 2017;650:60–4.
49. Preische O, Schultz SA, Apel A, et al. Serum neurofilament dynamics predicts neurodegeneration and clinical progression in presymptomatic Alzheimer's disease. Nat Med 2019;25(2):277–83.

Confounders in the Interpretation of Paraneoplastic and Neuronal Autoantibody Panels

Naveen George, DO, MHSA[a,b], Neel Fotedar, MD[a,b], Hesham Abboud, MD, PhD[a,b,*]

KEYWORDS

- Paraneoplastic • Neuronal autoantibody • Autoimmune encephalitis

KEY POINTS

- With increasing use of paraneoplastic antibody panels, there has been an increase in clinically irrelevant (false positive) results leading to unnecessary workup.
- Review of the tools that can be used clinically to decide if a paraneoplastic panel is warranted.
- Multiple antibodies are associated with low clinical relevance.
- This review provides a clinically practical approach to the interpretation of paraneoplastic panels.

INTRODUCTION

Paraneoplastic neurologic syndromes are a group of autoimmune disorders characterized by variable combinations of central and peripheral nervous system dysfunction secondary to an aberrant immune response targeting onconeuronal antigens.[1] Through a predominantly T-cell–mediated response, the immune system attacks nerve cells that harbor antigens with molecular resemblance to specific proteins in a known or developing neoplasm in the body.[2] As a byproduct of this immune response, several neuronal autoantibodies (NAAs) are formed serving as markers for paraneoplastic neuronal autoimmunity despite not being pathogenic themselves in most cases. These classical yet not pathogenic NAAs target intracellular antigens and include antineuronal nuclear Ab, type 1 (ANNA1 or anti-Hu), antineuronal nuclear Ab, type 2 (ANNA2 or anti-Ri), antineuronal nuclear Ab, type 3 (ANNA3), antiglial

[a] Multiple Sclerosis and Neuroimmunology Program, Neurological Institute, University Hospitals Cleveland Medical Center, 11100 Euclid Avenue, Cleveland, OH 44106, USA; [b] Case Western Reserve University School of Medicine, Cleveland, OH, USA
* Corresponding author. 11100 Euclid Avenue, Cleveland, OH 44106.
E-mail address: Hesham.Abboud@uhhospitals.org

Clin Lab Med 40 (2020) 305–316
https://doi.org/10.1016/j.cll.2020.05.004
0272-2712/20/© 2020 Elsevier Inc. All rights reserved.

nuclear Ab, type 1 (AGNA1), Purkinje cell cytoplasmic Ab, type 1 (PCAB1 or anti-Yo), Purkinje cell cytoplasmic Ab, type 2 (PCAB2), Purkinje cell cytoplasmic Ab, type Tr (PCATR), amphiphysin Ab (AMPH), and collapsin response mediator protein 5 (CRMP-5-IgG or anti-CV2).

A second category of paraneoplastic antibodies are directed against neuronal or muscular synaptic or ion channel antigens and can mediate a pathogenic humoral immune reaction that often results in a neuromuscular (neuropathic and/or myasthenic) syndrome depending on the specific antibody. These antibodies include P/Q-type calcium channel Ab (PQ-VGCC), N-type calcium channel Ab (N-VGCC), acetyl choline receptor (muscle) binding Ab (ACR-B), acetyl choline receptor (muscle) modulating Ab (ACR-M), acetyl choline receptor ganglionic neuronal Ab (ACR-G), neuronal voltage-gated potassium channel Ab (VGKC), and striational antibodies. Both paraneoplastic antibody categories are linked to specific types of neoplasms, most commonly small cell lung cancer (SCLC), breast cancer, thymic neoplasms, germ cell tumors, and lymphomas. The recent introduction of immune checkpoint inhibitors in the treatment of several types of advanced cancer has also resulted in novel paraneoplastic syndromes in patients with melanomas, renal cell carcinoma, and other unconventional cancers secondary to the heightened (unchecked) immune response.[3]

In addition to paraneoplastic intracellular and synaptic antibodies, a third and expanding category of pathogenic antibodies has evolved over the past decade, including antibodies directed against surface antigens strongly linked to autoimmune encephalitis.[4] These antibodies have variable rates of cancer association and are mostly non-paraneoplastic in origin. They mediate a form of autoimmune encephalitis that is more responsive to immunosuppressive therapy but has higher rates of recurrence compared with classical paraneoplastic syndromes. Examples of this expanding category include N-methyl-D-aspartate receptor Ab (NMDA-R), α-amino-3-hydroxy-5-methyl-4-isoxazolepropionic acid receptor Ab (AMPA-R), gamma-aminobutyric acid A receptor Ab (GABA-A-R), gamma-aminobutyric acid B receptor Ab (GABA-B-R), leucine-rich glioma inactivated Ab (LGI-1), and contactin-associated protein-like 2 Ab (CASPR2): the last 2 antibodies are part of the VGKC receptor complex. **Table 1** presents an overview of the clinical syndromes associated with the various categories of NAAs.

With the expansion of the available paraneoplastic and NAA panels and their increasing accessibility, concerns have been raised about their specificity and clinical relevance.[5] Rates of positive but clinically irrelevant paraneoplastic panels have been estimated to fall in the range of 60% to 70% based on patients who were initially thought to have a paraneoplastic or neuronal antibody-related syndrome but were eventually found to have a confirmed alternative diagnosis.[5,6] Literature has been published on untangling clinically relevant antibodies from clinically irrelevant antibodies, and various recommendations have been made by different investigators on how to properly interpret the results of these antibody panels when dealing with patients who might be suffering from paraneoplastic or non-paraneoplastic autoimmune neurologic syndromes.[5–7] In response to these concerns, large neuroimmunology laboratories have started to adopt a new model of testing that is symptom focused in order to overcome the problem of high false positive rates and improve the yield of testing.[8]

In this article, the authors review the various methods of testing for these antibodies, the literature published on the interpretation of the results of paraneoplastic and NAA antibody panels, and how the understanding of these results can be improved. Subsequently, this article discusses how a clinician can approach these results so as to optimize patient care.

Table 1
Paraneoplastic and non-paraneoplastic neurologic syndromes associated with neuronal auto antibodies

Antibody	Clinical/Anatomic Syndrome	Neurologic Presentation	Associated Tumor	% of Idiopathic Cases
1. Antibodies against intracellular antigens (classical onconeuronal antibodies)				
Hu (ANNA1)	PN, CD, LE, BE, CE	Sensory ataxia, pseudoathetosis, cerebellar ataxia, chorea, OMS	SCLC	2
Ri (ANNA2)	BE, CD	Ataxia, OMS, dystonia esp. jaw, chorea	Breast, SCLC	4
Yo (PCA1)	CD	Ataxia, tremor, chorea	Ovary, breast	2
CV2 (CRMP5)	SE, LE, CD, AIM, ON, CE	Chorea, NMO-like picture, ataxia, OMS, parkinsonism	SCLC, thymoma	4
Ma2	SE, LE, BE	Parkinsonism (PSP-like), ataxia, dystonia	Testicular seminoma	4
Tr/DNER	CD, LE	Ataxia	Hodgkin lymphoma	10
Amphiphysin	CE, AIM	Paraneoplastic SPS, PERM, myoclonus, hyperekplexia	Breast, SCLC	5
GAD65	CE, AIM, LE, CD	Idiopathic SPS, ataxia, seizures	Rarely thymoma	75
2. Antibodies against neuromuscular and ganglionic synaptic receptors				
PQ-VGCC	LEMS, PN, CD	LEMS, ataxia, neuropathy,	SCLC	79 (less in LEMS)
N-VGCC	LEMS, PN, CD	LEMS, ataxia, neuropathy	SCLC	79
Striational	Neuromuscular junction	Myasthenia gravis	Thymoma	Variable but high thymoma association if presenting with myasthenia
ACHR-B	Neuromuscular junction	Myasthenia gravis	Thymoma	10
ACHR-G	Ganglionopathy	Dysautonomia	Idiopathic	Majority are idiopathic

(continued on next page)

Table 1
(continued)

3. Antibodies against surface antigens

Antibody	Clinical/Anatomic Syndrome	Neurologic Presentation	Associated Tumor	% of Idiopathic Cases
NMDA	LE, CE, SE	Psychosis/AMS, speech dysfunction, orofacial dyskinesia, stereotypies, chorea, dystonia, catatonia, coma, seizures, dysautonomia	Ovarian teratoma or rarely testicular	41 (especially children)
AMPA	LE	Psychosis/AMS, seizures	SCLC, breast, thymoma	30
GABA-A	CE, AIM	SPS, seizures, status epilepticus	Thymoma	95
GABA-B	LE	Psychosis/AMS, seizures, status epilepticus	SCLC	50
Glycine R	Myelitis	SPS, PERM, hyperekplexia	Idiopathic	97
mGluR1/anti-Homer-3	CD	Ataxia	Hodgkin	Mostly paraneoplastic
mGluR5	LE	Ophelia syndrome	Hodgkin	Mostly paraneoplastic
VGKC (CASPR2)	LE, PN	Isaac syndrome: Myokymia, neuromyotonia, Morvan syndrome, myoclonus, chorea, CJD-like	Rare: thymoma, SCLC	70
VGKC (LGI1)	LE, SE	Faciobrachial dystonic seizures, ataxia, chorea, hyponatremia	Rare: thymoma, SCLC	70
DPPX	CE, dysautonomia	Hyperekplexia, myoclonus, seizures, AMS, diarrhea	Rare: lymphoma	90
D2	SE (pediatric basal ganglia encephalitis)	Parkinsonism, dystonia, oculogyric crisis, chorea	Idiopathic	100

Abbreviations: AIM, autoimmune myelitis; AMS, altered mental status; BE, brainstem encephalitis; CD, cerebellar degeneration; CE, cortical/subcortical encephalitis; CJD, Creutzfeldt-Jacob disease; LE, limbic encephalitis; NMO, neuromyelitis optica; OMS, opsoclonus myoclonus syndrome; ON, optic neuritis; PERM, progressive encephalomyelitis with rigidity and myoclonus; PN, peripheral neuropathy; PSP, progressive supranuclear palsy; SE, striatal encephalitis; SPS, stiff person syndrome.

DETECTION OF AUTOANTIBODIES: METHODS

The various methods available to detect these antibodies include immunohistochemistry/indirect immunofluorescence assay (IHC/IFA), Western blot, radioimmunoprecipitation assay (RIA), enzyme-linked immunosorbent assay, and cell-based assay (CBA).

Detection of classic onconeuronal antibodies and antibodies against neuronal surface antigens is slightly different because of the different location of the antigens. Also, onconeuronal antibodies mostly target linear epitopes, whereas surface antibodies mostly target conformational epitopes.[9]

Immunohistochemistry/Indirect Immunofluorescence Assay

Tissue-based assays use IHC/IFA to detect antibodies present in serum or cerebrospinal fluid (CSF) and can be used as the initial test to screen for both intracellular (type 1) and neuronal surface antibodies (type 2).[2] If using a rat brain, about 5- to 9-μm-thick slices are used,[9] but different pretreatment methods are required to detect type I and II antibodies. If using for group I antibodies, sliced brain tissue can be fixed with acetone or paraformaldehyde (PFA), whereas for group II antibodies, rat brain is first fixed with PFA, then cryoprotected with 40% sucrose for 24 hours, and then sliced using a cryostat.[9]

Following the pretreatment of the slices (cerebellum for group I and hippocampus for group II),[2] slices are incubated with the patient's specimen: CSF or serum, and stained with diaminobenzidine or fluorescently labeled antibodies to visualize the bound antibodies.[9]

Radioimmunoprecipitation Assay

RIA is used to detect group II antibodies, but if the surface channel has different components, then RIA might not be able to detect the individual components, for example, antibodies against VGKC complex proteins.[9]

Cell-Based Assay

CBAs detect antibodies based on expression of antigens on suitable cell lines transfected with a plasmid encoding the antigen.[2] Commercially available CBAs use human embryonic kidney cells, but there are other cell lines available as well. CBAs are used as confirmatory tests for group II antibodies.[2] CBAs can be live-cell or fixed-cell based. There is only 1 retrospective study that has compared the 2 techniques, and it commented that CBA with live cells actually had less specificity than CBA with fixed cells in patients with anti-NMDA-R encephalitis.[10]

In fixed-cell CBA, transfected cells are fixed with 4% PFA for 5 minutes at room temperature, permeabilized with 0.3% Triton X-100 for 5 minutes at room temperature, and then incubated with patient's serum or CSF for 2 hours at room temperature. In live-cell CBA, the live transfected cells are incubated with patient's serum for 1 hour at room temperature, followed by fixation and permeabilization.[10]

It should also be noted that for both fixed and live-cell CBAs, presence of the receptor on the membrane leaves them susceptible to excitotoxicity, so often receptor blockers are added to the culture medium, for example, ketamine for anti-NMDA-R antibodies.[9]

CBA analysis is user dependent because it requires a subjective visual scoring system with epifluorescent microscopy; most of the laboratories use 2 independent blinded observers to decrease error.[9] Because of this factor, IHC with serial dilutions has been found to be more sensitive to assess antibody titers during the course of the illness.[10]

One of the alternatives to make CBA more quantitative without using serial IHC dilutions for antibody titers is to use CBA with fluorescence activated cell sorting.[9]

SENSITIVITY AND SPECIFICITY OF ANTIBODY DETECTION METHODS

Various studies have been published commenting on sensitivity and specificity of various antibody detection methods for the specific antibodies. In general, permeabilized CBAs have higher sensitivity for CSF testing in conditions whereby there is increased intrathecal antibody production, for example, anti-NMDA-R antibodies, anti-AMPA-R antibodies, and anti-GABA-B-R antibodies.[9]

As an example, for anti-NMDA-R antibodies, a retrospective analysis done by Gresa-Arribas and colleagues[10] in 2014 on samples from 250 patients with anti-NMDA-R encephalitis (and 100 controls) showed that the sensitivity of IHC was 100% for CSF and 91.6% for serum. Sensitivity of fixed CBA was 100% for CSF and 86.8% for serum. They also assessed combined IHC and fixed CBA sensitivity and specificity. Combined sensitivity for CSF was 100%, and for serum, it was 85.6%. Combined specificity, on the other hand, for both CSF and serum was 100%.

CLINICAL CONCERNS WITH NEURONAL AUTOANTIBODY PANELS

The expansion in the number of recognized autoimmune/paraneoplastic antibodies and associated syndromes has led to a dramatic increase in the frequency of testing, and as a result, an increase in the number of seropositive cases.[4] Consequently, further investigation into the utility of the paraneoplastic and related NAA panels has ensued. The Mayo Clinic Neuroimmunology Laboratory offers some of the most commonly used and discussed NAA panels, which include 17 disease-specific profiles, 11 of which were launched since 2014.[8] One of the earliest and most commonly used Mayo panels is the Mayo Paraneoplastic Panel (Mayo Medical Laboratories Test ID: PAVAL), which is a cause-driven panel that can be tested in the serum or CSF. It has been debated that because of the large number of antibodies checked with the Mayo Clinic Paraneoplastic Panel, some of which involve the central nervous system, whereas others involve the peripheral nervous system, there is a high chance of clinically irrelevant results that can lead to unnecessary downstream testing, including avoidable computed tomographic scans, PET scans, or even biopsies.[5] Newer antibody panels from the same laboratory include most of the surface NAAs, which were only partially available as reflex tests in the original PAVAL panel. These NAAs against surface antigens are more likely to be clinically relevant especially in patients presenting with a picture suggestive of autoimmune encephalitis. Adopting a symptom-driven rather than a cause-driven approach when selecting an NAA panel is recommended by the laboratory to improve the yield of testing.[8] Several panels are currently available commercially, including panels for autoimmune encephalopathy (test ID: ENS1 and ENC1), movement disorders (test ID: MDS2 and MDC2), epilepsy (test ID: EPS1 and EPC1), and myelopathy (test ID: MAS1 and MAC1), available for both serum and CSF testing. The differences between these panels, however, are small and limited to 1 or 2 antibodies. Also, the wide syndromic overlap between the different antibodies makes it more practical to use the most comprehensive panel especially for vague or atypical cases. Other neuroimmunology laboratories offer similar panels that include a mixture of both highly clinically relevant and less clinically relevant antibodies. Perhaps the best clinical approach is one that reserves testing for cases with high pretest probability followed by critical evaluation of positive results to determine clinical relevance, as detailed later in this article.

ANTIBODIES WITH LOW CLINICAL RELEVANCE

Given the inherent risk that is involved when unclear or unexpected results occur with respect to the paraneoplastic panel, it is important to critically examine the utility in testing each of the antibodies on the panel. Five antibodies have been called into question as to their risk of producing clinically irrelevant (false positive) results.

Anti-Voltage-Gated Calcium Channel

Two such antibodies discussed were the P/Q and the N-type voltage-gated calcium channel (VGCC) antibodies.[5] Antibodies to the P/Q type VGCC have been reported to be the cause of Lambert-Eaton Myasthenic syndrome (LEMS) and have been associated with SCLC.[11] On further evaluation, however, it was noted in 1 retrospective study that most patients (58 out of 100) with positive VGCC-Ab titers did not have an autoimmune or inflammatory cause for their neurologic condition. In addition, there was shown to be a low specificity (36.17% for P/Q type and 65.96% for N-type) for the diagnosis of LEMS.[11] Of note, 67% of the cohort did not have cancer, which raises the question as to whether the presence of this autoimmune serologic marker should be used to guide further cancer screening.[11] There was also no difference in antibody titers between patients with clinically relevant and those with clinically irrelevant anti-VGCC antibodies or between those with cancer and those without cancer.[11] This in combination with the fact that there are comparable rates of positivity in populations with neurologic symptoms, healthy controls, and those who are neurologically asymptomatic, makes it difficult to judge if this antibody is directly involved with malignancy or paraneoplastic syndromes.[5]

Anti-Voltage-Gated Potassium Channel

The classic VGKC antibody syndromes are linked to antibodies directed to VGKC receptor complex proteins, namely anti-LGI-1 and anti-CASPR2. Anti-LGI-1 is often associated with classic limbic encephalitis and faciobrachial dystonic seizures, whereas CASPR2 is more often associated with Morvan syndrome, neuromyotonia, and dysautonomia.[12] Conversely, non-LGI-1 non-CASPR2 (double seronegative) anti-VGKC antibodies are of questionable clinical significance.[13] Studies before the wide availability of anti-LGI-1 and anti-CASPR2 antibodies suggested a role of anti-VGKC titer in determining clinical significance with quoted sensitivity and specificity for clinical relevance of 90% and 78.6%, respectively, if the titer was greater than 0.25 nM.[14] When the titer is less than 0.25 nM, the clinical relevance is limited.[12] However, in a more recent study that looked specifically at double seronegative anti-VGKC antibody-positive patients, antibody titers did not differ between those with antibodies that were deemed clinically relevant (28% of the cohort) and those with antibodies deemed irrelevant. Higher antibody titers were found mainly in patients with anti-LGI1 or anti-CASPR2 antibodies, suggesting that the value of anti-VGKC antibody titer from earlier studies was likely driven by patients who could have been positive to one of the VGKC protein complex antibodies but were not formally tested. Overall, in modern practice, patients with double seronegative anti-VGKC antibodies require detailed evaluation of clinical and ancillary data along with careful exclusion of other competing causes before attributing the neurologic presentation to the anti-VGKC antibody.

Antiganglionic Acetylcholine Receptor Antibody

A third antibody of low clinical relevance is the ganglionic acetylcholine receptor antibody (ACR-G-Ab).[5] The most closely associated syndrome linked with this antibody is autoimmune autonomic ganglionopathy (AAG), which is described as an immune-mediated disorder characterized by autonomic failure with dysfunction of the sympathetic, parasympathetic, and enteric nervous systems; however, this antibody also has associations with postural orthostatic tachycardia syndrome, small-fiber neuropathy, large-fiber neuropathy, and nonneurologic disorders like Sjögrens, celiac disease, and systemic lupus erythematosis.[15] In a retrospective study, only 22% of ACR-G-Ab-positive patients were found to have clinical AAG.[15] The presence of ACR-G-Ab without autonomic symptoms may reflect a nonspecific autoimmune response, as is the case with other antibodies previously discussed; however, it is clear that ACR-G-Ab plays an essential role in the pathogenesis of AAG because serum titers correlate with disease severity, and treatment with plasma exchange appears to lead to improvement.[15] It is suspected that the reason for the wide clinical spectrum associated with ACR-G-Ab is because the targeted subunit is distributed throughout the nervous system and is not confined to the autonomic ganglia.[15]

Anti-GAD65

Low titers of Anti-glutamic acid decarboxylase 65(GAD65) antibodies are often clinically irrelevant in patients with neurologic presentations and are linked more to propensity to type 1 diabetes and thyrogastric autoimmune disorders.[16] On the contrary, high titers of this antibody are often clinically relevant and are strongly associated with stiff person syndrome, cerebellar ataxia, autoimmune epilepsy, and/or limbic encephalitis.[6]

Striational Muscle Antibodies

Striational muscle antibodies have frequent clinically irrelevant results, and it is unclear which neurologic presentations are associated with the antibody other than myasthenia gravis for which other antibodies are better at identifying.[5]

NEURONAL AUTOANTIBODIES WITH HIGH CLINICAL RELEVANCE

Antibodies against intracellular antigens (classical onconeuronal antibodies category 1) are, in general, considered clinically relevant in patients with neurologic syndromes and are often predictive of associated cancer.[17] Likewise, antibodies against surface antigens associated with autoimmune encephalitis (category 3) are often clinically relevant when positive. One study that looked at the clinical relevance of serum anti-NMDA-R antibodies found that 77% of patients with anti-NMDA-R antibody have clinically relevant disease regardless of titer.[18]

CLINICAL SCALES

The *Antibody Prevalence-in Epilepsy and Encephalopathy Score (APE²)* (**Table 2**) has been developed as a tool to help identify patients expected to have positive NAA panel. By identifying multiple common factors that are commonly seen with autoimmune/paraneoplastic pathologic condition, this scale boasts a high statistical likelihood that a neural-specific autoantibody will be present. With a score greater than 3, it is 99% sensitive and 93% specific ($P < .0001$) in regards to identifying neural-specific antibodies. Furthermore, it has been proposed that this scale could be used in the diagnostic criteria of autoimmune encephalopathy in that an APE² score greater than 3 is "possible" autoimmune encephalopathy, an APE² score greater than 3 with positive neural specific antibody is "antibody positive" autoimmune encephalopathy, and an APE² score greater than 3 with a successful treatment with immunotherapy or an APE² score greater than 6 is "probable" autoimmune encephalopathy.[19]

Table 2
Antibody prevalence in epilepsy and encephalopathy

	Value
New onset, rapidly progressive mental status changes that developed over 1–6 wk or new onset seizure activity (within 1 y of evaluation)	1
Neuropsychiatric changes; agitation, aggressiveness, emotional lability	1
Autonomic dysfunction (sustained atrial tachycardia or bradycardia, orthostatic hypotension [at least 20 mm Hg decrease in systolic pressure of at least 10 mm Hg decrease in diastolic pressure within 3 min of quiet standing], hyperhidrosis, persistently labile blood pressure, ventricular tachycardia, cardiac asystole, or gastrointestinal dysmotility)	1
Viral prodrome (rhinorrhea, sore throat, low-grade fever) to be scored in the absence of underlying systemic malignancy within 5 y of neurologic symptom onset	2
Faciobrachial dystonic seizures	3
Facial dyskinesias, to be scored in the absence of faciobrachial dystonic seizures	2
Seizure refractory to at least 2 antiseizure medications	2
CSF findings consistent with inflammation (CSF protein >50 mg/dL, and/or lymphocytic pleocytosis >5 cells/µL, if the total number of CSF red blood cell count is <1000 cells/µL)	2
Brain MRI suggesting encephalitis (T2/fluid-attenuated inversion recovery hyperintensity restricted to one or both medial temporal lobes, or multifocal in gray matter, white matter, or both compatible with demyelination or inflammation)	2
Systemic cancer diagnosed within 5 y of neurologic symptom onset (excluding cutaneous squamous cell carcinoma, basal cell carcinoma, brain tumor, cancer with brain metastasis)	2

Adapted from Dubey D, Kothapalli N, McKeon A, et al. Predictors of neural-specific autoantibodies and immunotherapy response in patients with cognitive dysfunction. J Neuroimmunol. 2018;323:63; with permission.

The *Neuronal Autoantibody Confidence Scale (NACS)* (**Table 3**) was created to predict the clinical relevance of positive antibodies found via the serum paraneoplastic panel. Given the high rates of clinically irrelevant results often associated with the serum paraneoplastic panel, it is prudent to clarify the significance of antibody

Table 3
Neuronal autoantibody confidence scale

	Value
Antibody against intracellular antigens	1
Movement disorder and/or stiff person syndrome	1
Cancer and/or smoking history	1
Inflammatory CSF (either high cell count, IgG index, and/or positive OCBs)	1
Hyponatremia	1
Chronic course (>3 mo)	−1

IgG, immunoglobulin G; OCBs, oligoclonal bands.
Adapted from Abboud H, Rossman I, Mealy MA, et al. Neuronal autoantibodies: differentiating clinically relevant and clinically irrelevant results. J Neurol. 2017;264(11):2284–92; with permission.

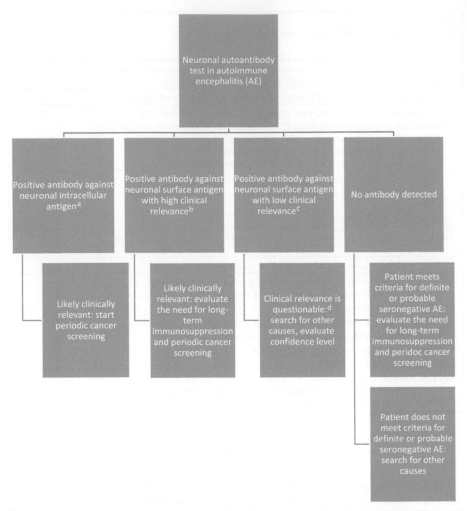

Fig. 1. Interpretation of the neuronal autoantibody panel. [a] Anti-Hu (ANNA-1), anti-Ri (ANNA-2), ANNA-3, anti-SOX1 (AGNA), anti-amphiphysin, anti-CRMP-5 (anti-CV2), anti-Yo (PCA-1), PCA-2, high-titer anti-GAD65. [b] Anti-NMDA-R, anti-LGI1, anti-CASPR2, anti-AMPA-R, anti-GABA-A/B, PCA-Tr, anti-DPPX, anti-mGluR1, anti-mGluR2, anti-mGluR5, anti-IgLON5, anti-AQP4, anti-MOG. [c] Non-LGI1 non-CASPR2 anti-VGKC, anti-P/Q VGCC, anti-N VGCC, Ach-b, Ach-M, Ach-G, Striational. [d] Low-titer anti-GAD65 is an antibody against cytoplasmic antigen but is of questionable clinical significance.

positivity and help guide the clinical decision making in regards to initiation of immunotherapy and periodic cancer screening. If a score greater than 1 is attained, it is likely that the antibody is clinically relevant (odds ratio [OR] 50.4, 95% confidence interval [CI; 8.2, 309.9], $P<.0001$), which is to say that the patient likely has an autoimmune/paraneoplastic neurologic syndrome related to the antibody. Conversely, if a score less than 1 is attained, it is likely that the antibody is clinically irrelevant (OR 42.7, CI [4.9, 370.2], $P = .0007$), whereas a score of 1 is not predictive.[6]

It is to be noted that the APE[2] score is meant to predict positivity to one or more NAAs, thus helping the clinician select cases for paraneoplastic and neuronal antibody panel testing in the acute setting, whereas the NACS score aids in the proper interpretation of positive results and selection of cases for periodic cancer screening and/or maintenance immunosuppression if indicated. Both scales are relatively recent and will require validation in different cohorts and likely several modifications before they are fully useable in the clinical setting.

SUMMARY

With the increasing recognition of paraneoplastic/autoimmune syndromes, there has been a dramatic increase in antibody testing via the paraneoplastic and related neuronal antibody panels.[6] Of concern, however, as with any diagnostic testing, is the chance for false positives and clinically irrelevant results that can arise leading to unnecessary worry, potentially invasive workup, and overall increased cost.[5] Further complicating the task is that the shifting sands inherent in the diagnosis of paraneoplastic syndromes, owing to the vagueness and commonality of usual symptoms, make positive antibody results more anomalous and an easy target to direct therapeutic attempts against. Misinterpretation of positive antibody panels might result in missing the true cause if the workup is halted consequent to the positive panel. It is for these reasons that the use of critical thinking by clinicians is of vital importance and that the ordering of paraneoplastic panels must be carried out judiciously and should be geared toward clinical manifestations and supported by typical findings on ancillary testing (eg, MRI, CSF).[7,20]

A practical approach to the interpretation of paraneoplastic and related NAA panels is presented in **Fig. 1**.

DISCLOSURE

Dr H. Abboud is a consultant for Biogen, Genentech, Sanofi Genzyme, Celgene, Alexion, and Viela Bio. He receives research support from Novartis, Genentech, and Celgene. The other authors have nothing to disclose.

REFERENCES

1. Lancaster E. Continuum: the paraneoplastic disorders. Continuum (Minneap Minn) 2015;21(2 0):452.

2. Höftberger R, Dalmau J, Graus F. Clinical neuropathology practice guide 5-2012: updated guideline for the diagnosis of anti-neuronal antibodies. Clin Neuropathol 2012;31(5):337.

3. Kumar N, Abboud H. Iatrogenic CNS demyelination in the era of modern biologics. Mult Scler 2019;25(8):1079–85.

4. Graus F, Titulaer MJ, Balu R, et al. A clinical approach to diagnosis of autoimmune encephalitis. Lancet Neurol 2016;15(4):391–404. https://doi.org/10.1016/S1474-4422(15)00401-9.

5. Ebright MJ, Li SH, Reynolds E, Burke JF, Claytor BR, Grisold A, Banerjee M, Callaghan BC. Unintended consequences of Mayo paraneoplastic evaluations. Neurology 2018;91(22):e2057–66. https://doi.org/10.1212/WNL.0000000000006577.

6. Abboud H, Rossman I, Mealy MA, Hill E, Thompson N, Banerjee A, Probasco J, Levy M. Neuronal autoantibodies: differentiating clinically relevant and clinically irrelevant results. J Neurol 2017;264(11):2284–92. https://doi.org/10.1007/s00415-017-8627-4.

7. Tebo AE, Haven TR, Jackson BR. Autoantibody diversity in paraneoplastic syndromes and related disorders: the need for a more guided screening approach. Clin Chim Acta 2016;459:162–9.

8. Pittock SJ, Mills JR, McKeon A. Reader response: unintended consequences of Mayo paraneoplastic evaluations. Neurology 2019;93(13):606.

9. van Coevorden-Hameete MH, Titulaer MJ, Schreurs MW, de Graaff E, Sillevis Smitt PA, Hoogenraad CC. Detection and characterization of autoantibodies to neuronal cell-surface antigens in the central nervous system. Front Mol Neurosci 2016;9:37. https://doi.org/10.3389/fnmol.2016.00037.

10. Gresa-Arribas N, Titulaer MJ, Torrents A, et al. Antibody titres at diagnosis and during follow-up of anti-NMDA receptor encephalitis: a retrospective study. Lancet Neurol 2014;13(2):167–77. https://doi.org/10.1016/S1474-4422(13)70282-5 [published correction appears in Lancet Neurol. 2014 Feb;13(2):135].

11. Di Lorenzo R, Mente K, Li J, et al. Low specificity of voltage-gated calcium channel antibodies in Lambert-Eaton myasthenic syndrome: a call for caution. J Neurol 2018;265(9):2114–9. https://doi.org/10.1007/s00415-018-8959-8.

12. Paterson RW, Zandi MS, Armstrong R, Vincent A, Schott JM. Clinical relevance of positive voltage-gated potassium channel (VGKC)-complex antibodies: experience from a tertiary referral centre. J Neurol Neurosurg Psychiatry 2014;85(6): 625–30. https://doi.org/10.1136/jnnp-2013-305218.

13. van Sonderen A, Schreurs MW, de Bruijn MA, et al. The relevance of VGKC positivity in the absence of LGI1 and Caspr2 antibodies. Neurology 2016;86(18): 1692–9. https://doi.org/10.1212/WNL.0000000000002637.

14. Jammoul A, Shayya L, Mente K, Li J, Rae-Grant A, Li Y. Clinical utility of seropositive voltage-gated potassium channel-complex antibody. Neurol Clin Pract 2016; 6(5):409–18. https://doi.org/10.1212/CPJ.0000000000000268.

15. Li Y, Jammoul A, Mente K, et al. Clinical experience of seropositive ganglionic acetylcholine receptor antibody in a tertiary neurology referral center. Muscle Nerve 2015;52(3):386–91. https://doi.org/10.1002/mus.24559.

16. Pittock SJ, Yoshikawa H, Ahlskog JE, et al. Glutamic acid decarboxylase autoimmunity with brainstem, extrapyramidal, and spinal cord dysfunction. Mayo Clin Proc 2006;81(9):1207–14. https://doi.org/10.4065/81.9.1207.

17. Dalmau J, Rosenfeld MR. Paraneoplastic syndromes of the CNS. Lancet Neurol 2008;7(4):327–40.

18. Zandi MS, Paterson RW, Ellul MA, et al. Clinical relevance of serum antibodies to extracellular N-methyl-D-aspartate receptor epitopes. J Neurol Neurosurg Psychiatry 2015;86(7):708–13. https://doi.org/10.1136/jnnp-2014-308736.

19. Dubey D, Kothapalli N, McKeon A, Flanagan EP, Lennon VA, Klein CJ, Britton JW, So E, Boeve BF, Tillema JM, Sadjadi R, Pittock SJ. Predictors of neural-specific autoantibodies and immunotherapy response in patients with cognitive dysfunction. J Neuroimmunol 2018 Oct 15;323:62–72. https://doi.org/10.1016/j.jneuroim.2018.07.009.

20. Callaghan BC, Burke JF. Author response: Unintended consequences of Mayo paraneoplastic evaluations. Neurology 2019;93(13):606–7. https://doi.org/10.1212/WNL.0000000000008180.

Reference Laboratory Testing for Neurologic Disorders

A. Zara Herskovits, MD, PhD*, Loren J. Joseph, MD

KEYWORDS

- Neurologic diseases • Send-out tests • Utilization review • Laboratory testing
- Cost containment

KEY POINTS

- The volume and variety of test requests received by the hospital clinical laboratory that are sent out for additional testing at reference laboratories have been increasing annually.
- Neurologic disease testing represents roughly 10% of the volume of tests sent to reference laboratories from our academic center.
- A variety of analytical methods are used for neurologic disease tests performed at reference laboratories, including mass spectrometry, nucleic acid testing, immunoassay, Western blot, and radioimmunoassay.
- Educational efforts, decision support, limiting orders, and active monitoring of requests have been used to facilitate the provision of high-quality, cost-effective laboratory services.

INTRODUCTION

Laboratory testing plays a critical role in the diagnosis and monitoring of patients with neurologic disorders. Although common tests are typically performed in a central hospital laboratory, an increasing number of essential but esoteric tests are sent to reference laboratories or other outside health care facilities. These assays often require specialized methodologies, interpretive expertise, or are infrequently ordered and therefore economically inefficient for a hospital laboratory to maintain.[1] Although having access to a broad test selection menu may help providers to establish a diagnosis and treatment plan, the negative consequences of sending tests to an outside facility include errors in test selection, problems with unfamiliar sample collection protocols, inaccurate result entry, turnaround time delays, and additional cost.[2,3]

Increases in the number and complexity of available laboratory tests can lead to suboptimal ordering patterns, including overuse (performing tests that are not

Department of Pathology, Beth Israel Deaconess Medical Center, 330 Brookline Avenue, Boston, MA 02215, USA
* Corresponding author.
E-mail address: aherskov@bidmc.harvard.edu

clinically indicated) and underuse (missing diagnostically important assays).[4] It is estimated that underuse occurs more frequently than overuse and may impact patient
care owing to missed diagnoses or delayed treatment.[5,6] Inappropriate laboratory
testing impacts patient care because it can trigger further diagnostic workups, referrals, and treatment that may not be necessary. Five percent of assay results are expected to be outside of the reference interval for test results that exhibit a normal
distribution, and it is likely that overuse increases the number of false negatives and
false positives that may require further medical attention.[7] Iatrogenic anemia can be
another negative consequence of inappropriate laboratory testing if excessive laboratory draws are performed, particularly in vulnerable populations such as neonatal and
critical care patients.[8–10]

Over the past decade, a number of advances have occurred in our understanding of
the pathophysiologic basis of neurologic disorders and several of these findings have
been translated into clinical diagnostic assays. Nucleic acid tests for spinal muscular
atrophy, epilepsy, frontotemporal dementia, and amyotrophic lateral sclerosis have
been developed[11–13]; however, their interpretation can be complex, incorporating
repeat expansions, point mutations, and copy number variants. Within the domain
of neuroimmunology, paraneoplastic syndrome and autoimmune encephalitis panels
that detect autoantibodies associated with motor dysfunction, seizures, memory loss,
vision problems, and other neurologic problems have become available.[14,15] These
genetic and immunologic testing panels are typically sent to reference laboratories
because they require specialized techniques and interpretive expertise.

In this article, we analyze recent trends in neurologic disease test requests that are
sent from our hospital laboratory to outside testing facilities. We also review practices
to improve operational efficiency such as use review, educational initiatives, decision
support, and limiting test orders. To illustrate how these strategies are practiced at our
institution, the ordering workflow for paraneoplastic panels and myasthenia gravis
testing is described in greater detail. These review practices are not only used for
neurologic disease testing, but also can be applied more broadly to other areas of laboratory medicine.

METHODS

This study was conducted at Beth Israel Deaconess Medical Center (BIDMC), a 673-
bed academic medical center in Boston, Massachusetts. At our institution, review of
selected tests sent to reference laboratories is performed by residents and attendings
from the chemistry, transfusion medicine, microbiology, hematology, cytology, molecular pathology, and neurology services. Neurologic disease testing is reviewed by attendings from the neurology or pathology services.

A retrospective analysis of neurologic disease testing was performed by querying
laboratory databases to analyze test requests sent from BIDMC to reference laboratories and other clinical testing sites between January 1, 2014, and December 31,
2018. Samples sent directly from outpatient provider offices to diagnostic testing
companies were not included in this analysis because this information was not accessible by central database searches of laboratory test requests. This project was sub-
mitted to the Institutional Review Board at BIDMC and was determined to be a quality
improvement project by the Committee on Clinical Investigations.

RESULTS

The overall volume of tests received by the central laboratory at BIDMC for analysis at
outside reference facilities has increased from 103,074 in 2014 to 130,895 tests in

2018 (**Fig. 1**A) and the number of different types of tests also increased during this time interval from 781 to 895 types of tests (**Fig. 1**B). In general, the fraction of neurologic disease testing comprised roughly 10% of the total number of assays sent to reference laboratories (**Fig. 2**A). In this analysis, neurologic disease testing was broadly defined to include assays for neurologic disorders (such as spinal muscular atrophy or Alzheimer's disease), toxic exposures with neurologic sequelae (such as lead poisoning), therapeutic drug monitoring (such as testing for levels of anticonvulsant medications), infectious diseases (such as JC virus), and deficient or excessive ingestion of vitamins and trace minerals (such as methylmalonic acid testing) that can impact the central or peripheral nervous system (**Fig. 2**B).

A more detailed breakdown of the major tests in each category indicates that multiple tests are often requested to assess the same condition. For example, the second most commonly ordered test for toxic exposures that can result in neurologic symptoms is the heavy metal screen, which tests for arsenic, lead, and mercury at the reference laboratory used at our institution[16]; however, lead and mercury are also frequently ordered as individual assays. In the nutrient excess or deficiency category, both methylmalonic acid and intrinsic factor antibody testing can be useful for diagnosis of vitamin B_{12} deficiency. Two complementary tests for syphilis (venereal disease research laboratory and fluorescent treponemal antibody tests) are among the most frequently ordered tests in the infectious disease testing category (**Table 1**).

Next, we analyzed the methods used for neurologic disease testing at reference laboratories to gain more perspective on the necessity of relying on outside facilities. We found that a variety of analytical techniques were used, with the greatest number of

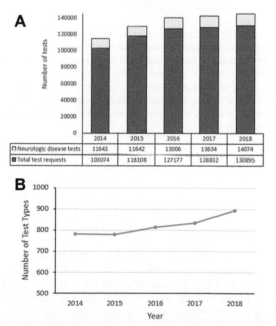

Fig. 1. Requests for reference laboratory testing received by the BIDMC central laboratory from 2014 to 2018. (*A*) Total number of tests requested annually and fraction of tests for neurologic disease testing. (*B*) Number of different types of tests requested by ordering providers to outside laboratories during each calendar year.

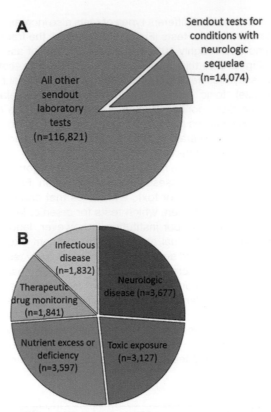

Fig. 2. Categories of reference laboratory test requests in 2018. (*A*) Test requests were categorized to determine the proportion of assays used to diagnose or monitor conditions with neurologic signs or symptoms. (*B*) Assays were further categorized into tests for neurologic disorders (such as spinal muscular atrophy or Alzheimer's disease); toxic exposures with neurologic sequelae (such as lead poisoning); vitamin and nutrient excess or deficiency (such as methylmalonic acid levels); therapeutic drug monitoring (such as testing for levels of anticonvulsant medications) and infectious diseases that can impact the central or peripheral nervous system (such as JC virus).

tests performed with mass spectrometry. Roughly one-half of these mass spectrometry test requests were for the identification of inorganic compounds such as heavy metals and 30% were assays for vitamins and trace minerals. Therapeutic monitoring of drugs such as leviracetam or lamotrigine comprised most of the remaining 20% of these requests (data not shown). Other commonly used test methodologies include nucleic acid testing, immunoassays, Western blot, radioimmunoprecipitation assays, immunofluorescence, or a combination of techniques (**Fig. 3**).

Several strategies for improving the efficiency of laboratory test ordering were identified based on the literature and an evaluation of the methods used at our institution (**Fig. 4**). These techniques include educational initiatives, decision support, active monitoring, and cost control measures. To underscore how these strategies can be applied, the ordering workflow for paraneoplastic/encephalopathy panels and myasthenia gravis testing at our institution were analyzed in greater detail.

Encephalitis is an inflammatory brain condition that can be caused by antibodies against neuronal or synaptic proteins. In paraneoplastic syndrome cases, neurologic

Table 1
The 5 most commonly ordered neurologic disease tests within each testing category (neurologic disorders, toxic exposures, vitamin or nutrient excess or deficiency, therapeutic drug monitoring, or infectious diseases)

Test Name	Number of Tests (2018)
Neurologic disease	
Spinal muscular atrophy carrier testing	1077
JC virus antibody with reflex to inhibition assay	568
Ceruloplasmin	325
Paraneoplastic autoantibody evaluation	217
Acetylcholine receptor antibody	169
Toxic exposures	
Lead	2905
Heavy metal screen	134
Mercury	69
Cobalt	5
Aluminum	5
Nutrient excess or deficiency	
Methylmalonic acid	1670
Copper	680
Vitamin B_1	421
Vitamin E	228
Intrinsic factor antibody	205
Therapeutic drug monitoring	
Levetiracetam	544
Lamotrigine	467
Lacosamide	168
Trileptal	141
Zonisamide	137
Infectious disease testing	
Lyme disease antibody, immunoblot	479
Herpes simplex virus, polymerase chain reaction	349
Varicella DNA, polymerase chain reaction	205
Venereal disease research laboratory (VDRL)	93
Fluorescent treponemal antibody (FTA-ABS)	76

symptoms are associated with malignancies. Clinicians frequently request paraneoplastic and encephalitis antibody panels, which are complex groups of laboratory tests that have a significant number of common assays, such ganglionic acetylcholine receptor (AchR) or amphiphysin antibody assays (**Fig. 5**).[17,18] At our hospital, neurologists or pathologists review these test requests to evaluate whether ordering these large testing panels is clinically justified. Technologists in the central hospital laboratory also play a role in limiting test orders by canceling one panel request when paraneoplastic and encephalopathy panels are ordered on the same patient at the same time. The second panel can be performed subsequently in circumstances when it is clinically indicated.

An analysis of test use patterns for the paraneoplastic panel indicate that test requests have increased by more than 5-fold between 2014 and 2018 (**Fig. 6**A) with

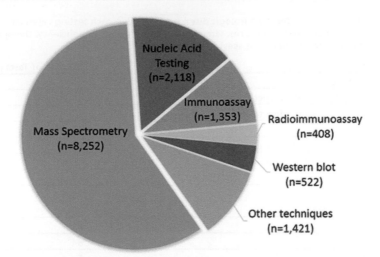

Fig. 3. Methodologies used for neurologic disease tests performed at reference laboratories. Tests requested in 2018 from the BIDMC central laboratory were categorized by analytical techniques used.

the majority of test requests coming from the neurology service (**Fig. 6**B). Over a 5-year period, roughly 2.5% of tests were canceled owing to the overlap in testing when providers sent requests for both paraneoplastic testing and encephalopathy assays on the same patient at the same time. A similar fraction of tests were canceled by

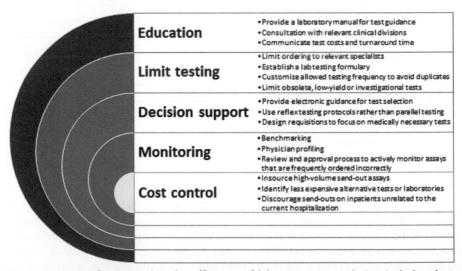

Fig. 4. Strategies for improving the efficiency of laboratory test ordering include educational initiatives (such as providing a laboratory manual to guide best practices for test ordering), limiting testing (either to certain groups of providers or under certain circumstances where the assays or likely to be low yield), decision support (including electronic pop-ups or other guidance provided as the provider is placing the order), active monitoring (including review and approval for tests that are frequently ordered incorrectly), and cost control measures (such as identifying less expensive alternative assays or reference laboratories).

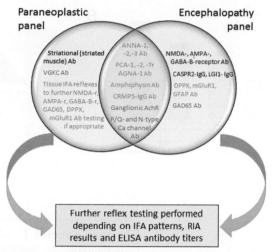

Fig. 5. Comparison of paraneoplastic and encephalopathy panel reference laboratory testing. Abbreviation for assays used in the Venn diagram are: AchR, acetylcholine receptor; AGNA, anti-glial/neuronal nuclear antibody; AMPA-r, alpha-amino-3-hydroxy-5-methyl-4-isoxazolepropionic acid receptor; ANNA, antineuronal nuclear antibody-type; CASPR2, contactin-associated protein-like 2; CRMP5, collapsin response-mediator protein 5 neuronal; DPPX, dipeptidyl-peptidase-like protein 6; GABA-B-r, gamma-aminobutyric acid-B receptor; GAD, glutamic acid decarboxylase; GFAP, glial fibrillary acidic protein alpha subunit; LGI1, leucine-rich glioma inactivated 1; mGluR1, metabotropic glutamate receptor; NMDA-r, *N*-methyl-ᴅ-aspartate receptor; PCA, Purkinje cell cytoplasmic antibody; VGKC, voltage-gated potassium channel. Enzyme linked immunosorbent assays (ELISA) are depicted in *black*, immunofluorescence (IFA) tests are shown in *green*, radioimmunoprecipitation assay (RIA) in *blue*, and cell-based assays (CBA) in *red*. This schematic reflects tests performed at Mayo Medical Laboratories.[17,18]

providers or the neurology service after review of the test's usefulness relative to the patient's presentation and clinical data (**Fig. 6**C).

Serologic testing for myasthenia gravis is an example of how decision support can be applied centrally to improve testing efficiency. Myasthenia gravis is a neuromuscular disorder characterized by episodic muscular weakness caused by an autoimmune response against the neuromuscular junction and serologic testing is an important component of diagnosis (**Fig. 7**). A number of postsynaptic membrane proteins including the AchR, muscle-specific tyrosine kinase (MuSK), and low-density lipoprotein receptor-related 4 can be targeted during the disease process. The number of requests for MuSK assays have increased between 2013 and 2018 (**Fig. 8**A), with the majority of the test requests coming from the neurology service (**Fig. 8**B). Because 90% of patients with generalized myasthenia are AchR positive, they do not require MuSK or other testing for diagnosis. Therefore, requests for MuSK testing are canceled by our clinical laboratory when a patient has a positive AchR test result. This reflexing strategy has a greater impact on canceling unnecessary laboratory testing relative to active monitoring (**Fig. 8**C).

DISCUSSION

The use of diagnostic testing has increased rapidly throughout the world over the past several decades.[7,19] Interventions to decrease test order volume have been identified

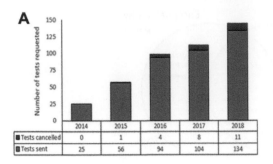

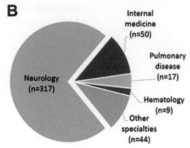

C

437 requests (5.5% canceled) for paraneoplastic antibody panels from 2014 to 2018

11 tests canceled (2.5%) due to overlapping testing with encephalopathy panel

9 tests canceled (2.1%) after pathologist or neurologist review

4 tests canceled (0.9%) by other providers

Fig. 6. Serum paraneoplastic antibody testing. (*A*) Tests requested annually between 2014 and 2018 with tests sent from the BIDMC central laboratory indicated in gray and tests canceled indicated in *red*. (*B*) Providers requesting paraneoplastic panels by department. (*C*) Number of tests canceled owing to repeat testing from overlap with encephalopathy panels and test auditing by pathologists or neurologists.

in a number of studies and tailoring these techniques to the appropriate clinical setting may decrease costs and improve operational efficiency for the laboratory.[20] Over the 5-year period analyzed in this article, the number of requests for reference laboratory testing increased by almost 28,000 tests and roughly 10% of these requests were for assays related to neurologic disease testing. In addition, the number of different diagnostic tests also increased during this period. These increases in both the volume of assay requests and types of tests not only impacts the laboratory budget, but also affects laboratory efficiency by increasing the amount of time required to audit these tests and communicate with ordering providers.

Although we did observe that multiple tests are often requested to assess the same condition, further analysis to evaluate the diagnostic yield and context of these test orders will be required before we can conclude whether these testing patterns are redundant or appropriate. For example, if requests for lead or mercury levels are used to follow a patient with prior abnormal results on a heavy metal screening panel, then the test requests may be appropriate. However, if both heavy metal screening and the individual tests that comprise this panel are ordered concurrently on the same patient, it may be a sign that provider education or active monitoring may be of benefit.

To gain more perspective on the necessity of relying on reference laboratories for an increasing number of specialty tests, analytical methods used for neurologic disease

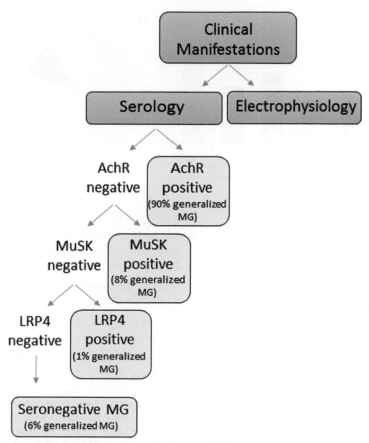

Fig. 7. Diagnostic testing for myasthenia gravis (MG). Testing may be initiated when a patient presents with clinical manifestations such as episodic weakness of ocular, limb, bulbar, or respiratory muscle groups. Electrophysiologic tests include repetitive nerve stimulation and single-fiber electromyography. Serologic assays include acetylcholine receptor (AchR) antibodies, muscle-specific tyrosine kinase (MuSK) antibodies, and low-density lipoprotein receptor-related 4 (LRP4) antibodies.

send-outs were tabulated to assess the possibility of insourcing. We found that the majority of tests were performed with mass spectrometry; however, it is worth noting that the methodologies are not uniform. For example, induction coupled mass spectrometry was performed to detect heavy metals, whereas liquid chromatography with tandem mass spectrometry was used to assess levels of anticonvulsant medications from patient samples. Because different separation strategies, ionization techniques, and analyzers can be used for mass spectrometry tests, insourcing of these assays must be evaluated in the context of expertise and instrumentation that is locally available.

We found that other commonly used methodologies for neurologic disease testing included nucleic acid testing, immunoassays, and immunofluorescence. Although the instrumentation to perform these techniques is available in our laboratory, the volume for some tests is not substantial enough for our hospital laboratories to maintain quality control and proficiency testing on a continual basis. In other cases, intellectual

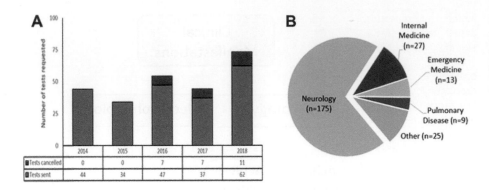

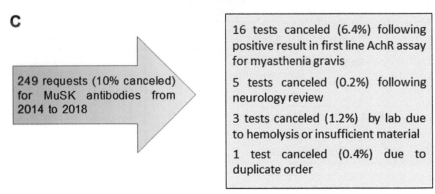

Fig. 8. Muscle-specific kinase (MuSK) autoantibody testing. (*A*) Tests requested annually between 2014 and 2018 with tests sent from the BIDMC central laboratory indicated in gray and the tests canceled in *red*. (*B*) Providers requesting MuSK testing by department. (*C*) Number and percentage of tests canceled owing to reflexive testing after positive result in first line testing, test auditing, specimen quality or quantity, or duplicate requests.

property and time required for our hospital laboratory to develop and maintain these specialty tests precludes insourcing. Therefore, many factors must be evaluated when considering whether testing can be brought in house.

A number of strategies including educational initiatives, decision support, active monitoring and cost control measures can be used for improving the efficiency of laboratory test ordering, and the optimal use of these approaches in a hospital setting may need additional study.[7] At our institution, we use a combination of these techniques, using pathology residents and attendings to actively monitor test use and working with clinical teams and laboratory information support staff to guide order entry.

One of the challenges in using educational interventions is the high level of turnover of house staff in an academic teaching hospital. Roughly one-third of medicine and pediatric residents turn over annually,[20] which means that didactic approaches involving presentations or emails may not have a long-lasting institutional impact unless senior-level physicians are able to reinforce test use practices continuously. Providing an online laboratory manual is one of the strategies used to educate clinical providers at our institution. This web-based test menu includes information about the purpose of the assay, specimen requirements, turnaround times, and reference intervals. This document can also be used to guide best practices for test ordering by including information about test cost, interpretation, and clinical settings where the assay may or may not be indicated.[10] External links to practice guidelines from professional societies and reference laboratory websites can also be provided.[10]

Setting limits on laboratory test ordering is another approach used to improve laboratory stewardship. The example provided elsewhere in this article describing how requests for paraneoplastic and encephalopathy panels are processed when they are requested simultaneously on the same patient is one way in which testing is restricted at our institution. This approach decreases redundant testing within diagnostic panels to improve cost efficiency. Another approach to limiting testing is the use of a laboratory testing formulary or clinical advisory committee that specifies a limited number of orderable tests and requires additional review for requests that are not on this predetermined list.[20–22] Because the number and complexity of medical tests is continually evolving, vetting new laboratory assays can require a substantial time commitment to understand whether the usefulness of an test is supported by evidence-based practice.[22]

Decision support and the use of computerized provider order entry can assist clinicians by providing information about a test as the provider is placing the order and can facilitate the use of reflex panels. In the example described, performing an initial AchR serology for patients with suspected myasthenia gravis and only reflexing those tests with a negative result for further testing is a more efficient testing strategy than performing all of the requested assays, resulting in the cancellation of 6.4% of MuSK tests relative to the 0.5% of tests canceled from active monitoring by the neurology service over a 5-year period.

Active monitoring of laboratory test requests is another strategy performed at many hospitals, including our own. In some cases, review and approval is required for tests that are over a certain cost threshold. At our institution and others,[4] tests that are not performed in the hospital laboratory and are frequently ordered incorrectly are also restricted, requiring approval from a pathologist or neurologist. Unfortunately, this review process can be time consuming and the number of tests canceled may be dwarfed by the increase in laboratory testing that occurs across an institution annually.

The importance of educating clinicians about test costs may need further study, because studies have found conflicting results on whether showing test charges at the time of ordering decreases the overuse of diagnostic testing.[23–26] Investigating whether there is a way to optimize price transparency so that it is both reproducible and sustainable may provide an important tool for cost containment in hospitals.

In this article, we have examined trends in neurologic disease test requests received by our hospital laboratory for assays performed at outside reference laboratories and reviewed strategies for improving the efficiency of our testing. Although our institution uses multiple methods to limit suboptimal test ordering practices, much more work remains to be done to optimize the quality, effectiveness, and usefulness of testing that is performed on patients seen at our hospital and its affiliated clinics.

SUMMARY

Suboptimal use of laboratory testing is an increasing problem common to neurologic disease testing and many other areas of laboratory medicine. Although the tests performed at outside laboratories comprise a small fraction of our overall volume, they represent a disproportionate share of the total laboratory costs. Combining educational efforts, decision support, limiting orders, active auditing, and other interventions are important elements for delivering high-quality, cost-effective laboratory services.

ACKNOWLEDGMENTS

The authors would like to thank Dr Lynne Uhl for her helpful comments and review of this article.

DISCLOSURE

The authors have nothing to disclose.

REFERENCES

1. Carter E, Bennett BD. Reference test review by pathology house staff: a cost-containment strategy for the clinical laboratory. Clin Leadersh Manag Rev 2002;16(1):3–6.
2. Dickerson JA, Cole B, Conta JH, et al. Improving the value of costly genetic reference laboratory testing with active utilization management. Arch Pathol Lab Med 2014;138(1):110–3.
3. Valenstein PN, Walsh MK, Stankovic AK. Accuracy of send-out test ordering: a college of American pathologists Q-probes study of ordering accuracy in 97 clinical laboratories. Arch Pathol Lab Med 2008;132(2):206–10.
4. Krasowski MD, Chudzik D, Dolezal A, et al. Promoting improved utilization of laboratory testing through changes in an electronic medical record: experience at an academic medical center. BMC Med Inform Decis Mak 2015;15(1):1–10.
5. Baird GS, Jackson BR, Dickerson J, et al. What's new in laboratory test utilization management? Clin Chem 2018;64(7):994–1000.
6. Zhi M, Ding EL, Theisen-Toupal J, et al. The landscape of inappropriate laboratory testing: a 15-year meta-analysis. PLoS One 2013;8(11):1–8.
7. Bindraban RS, ten Berg MJ, Naaktgeboren CA, et al. Reducing test utilization in hospital settings: a narrative review. Ann Lab Med 2018;38(5):402–12.
8. Jakacka N, Snarski E, Mekuria S. Prevention of iatrogenic anemia in critical and neonatal care. Adv Clin Exp Med 2016;25(1):191–7.
9. Signorelli H, Straseski JA, Genzen JR, et al. Benchmarking to identify practice variation in test ordering: a potential tool for utilization management. Lab Med 2015;46(4):356–64.
10. Lewandrowski K. Integrating decision support into a laboratory utilization management program. Clin Lab Med 2019;39(2):245–57.
11. Costain G, Cordeiro D, Matviychuk D, et al. Clinical application of targeted next-generation sequencing panels and whole exome sequencing in childhood epilepsy. Neuroscience 2019;418:291–310.
12. Renton AE, Majounie E, Waite A, et al. A hexanucleotide repeat expansion in C9ORF72 is the cause of chromosome 9p21-linked ALS-FTD. Neuron 2011;72(2):257–68.
13. DeJesus-Hernandez M, Mackenzie IR, Boeve BF, et al. Expanded GGGGCC hexanucleotide repeat in noncoding region of C9ORF72 causes chromosome 9p-linked FTD and ALS. Neuron 2011;72(2):245–56.
14. López-Chiriboga AS, Flanagan EP. Diagnostic and therapeutic approach to autoimmune neurologic disorders. Semin Neurol 2018;38(3):392–402.
15. Ebright MJ, Li SH, Reynolds E, et al. Unintended consequences of Mayo paraneoplastic evaluations. Neurology 2018;91(22):e2057–66.
16. Heavy metals panel, blood. Quest diagnostics. Available at: https://testdirectory.questdiagnostics.com/test/test-detail/7655/heavy-metals-panel-blood?cc=MASTER. Accessed December 17, 2019.

17. Paraneoplastic evaluation algorithm. Mayo clinic laboratories. Available at: https://www.mayocliniclabs.com/test-catalog/Overview/83380.   Accessed December 17, 2019.
18. Encephalopathy evaluation algorithm, Mayo clinic laboratories. Available at: https://www.mayocliniclabs.com/test-catalog/Clinical+and+Interpretive/92116. Accessed December 17, 2019.
19. van Walraven C, Naylor D. Do we now know what inappropriate laboratory utilization is? An expanded systematic review of laboratory clinical audits. JAMA 1998; 280(6):550–8.
20. Kim JY, Dzik WH, Dighe AS, et al. Utilization management in a large urban academic medical center: a 10-year experience. Am J Clin Pathol 2011;135(1): 108–18.
21. Harb R, Hajdasz D, Landry ML, et al. Improving laboratory test utilisation at the multihospital yale new haven health system. BMJ Open Qual 2019;8(3):e000689.
22. Warren JS. Laboratory test utilization program: structure and impact in a large academic medical center. Am J Clin Pathol 2013;139(3):289–97.
23. Feldman LS, Shihab HM, Thiemann D, et al. Impact of providing fee data on laboratory test ordering: a controlled clinical trial. JAMA Intern Med 2013;173(10): 903–8.
24. Horn DM, Koplan KE, Senese MD, et al. The impact of cost displays on primary care physician laboratory test ordering. J Gen Intern Med 2014;29(5):708–14.
25. Sedrak MS, Myers JS, Small DS, et al. Effect of a price transparency intervention in the electronic health record on clinician ordering of inpatient laboratory tests: the PRICE randomized clinical trial. JAMA Intern Med 2017;177(7):939–45.
26. Goetz C, Rotman SR, Hartoularos G, et al. The effect of charge display on cost of care and physician practice behaviors: a systematic review. J Gen Intern Med 2015;30(6):835–42.

The Development of New Diagnostic Tests for Neurologic Disorders in the Commercial Laboratory Environment

Iswariya Venkataraman, PhD, Stanley J. Naides, MD*

KEYWORDS

- Neuroimmunology • Neurodegeneration • Biomarker • Laboratory development
- Validation • Laboratory developed test

KEY POINTS

- Commercial laboratories are a highly regulated industry with oversight from federal and state governments and professional societies.
- Fundamental research to develop new diagnostic tests has shifted from commercial laboratories to academia, biotechnology startups, and a limited number of manufacturers.
- Outsourcing of early research and development limits financial risk, but may degrade in-house capabilities and add additional costs that offset outsourcing savings.
- Commercial laboratories must consider market readiness of a test, including target population size, medical provider acceptance, practice guidelines, and reimbursement environment.
- Commercial laboratories may provide decreased costs to patients and payers through economy of scale, improvements in high throughput testing, efficiencies in automation, and competition.

INTRODUCTION

Commercial laboratories are a highly regulated industry.[1] Oversight and guidelines for practices and procedures are provided by federal, state and, in many cases, local laws, statutes, and regulations.[2] In addition, professional societies in laboratory medicine provide practice guidelines and standards and certifications for laboratories and personnel. Testing performance is regularly audited through internal and external

Scientific Affairs, EUROIMMUN US, 1 Bloomfield Avenue, Mountain Lakes, New Jersey 07046, USA
* Corresponding author.
E-mail address: stanley.naides@euroimmun.us

Clin Lab Med 40 (2020) 331–339
https://doi.org/10.1016/j.cll.2020.06.001
0272-2712/20/© 2020 Elsevier Inc. All rights reserved.

proficiency programs. Federal and state programs, or their designees, regularly inspect and audit commercial laboratories.[3,4]

Development of new laboratory tests for neurologic disorders in a commercial laboratory environment is challenging scientifically, practically, commercially, and financially. New laboratory testing occasionally requires development of new methodology for detecting known biomarkers, but more often requires discovery of novel biomarkers. Transitioning a test performed in a research laboratory to a commercial laboratory environment typically necessitates test improvements for consistency, reliability, precision, and robustness. To be commercially viable, a test must be both acceptable and desired by the medical community. Predicting markets for a novel laboratory test is fraught by limited market research, unanswered questions about reimbursement, and often absent professional society guidelines on use of the testing. The cost to laboratories in acquiring intellectual property and reagents, performing assay development and validation, operationalizing a test, and preparing laboratory information systems and provider electronic medical records to receive results are all considerations in deciding to bring up and in offering a test.

IDENTIFYING A NEW TEST

Beginning in the 1980s, the pharmaceutical industry began downsizing in-house early pipeline research and development (R&D) and increasingly looked to outside sources for discovery and proof of concept, in order to minimize financial risk of early in-house development projects that fail. Instead, Pharma shifted to university sources for discovery, and as the biotechnology industry grew, increasingly looked to start-up venture capital to assume the risk.[5,6] This trend was also seen in the laboratory industry.[7]

Today, few commercial laboratories have an extensive research infrastructure to do discovery. The infrastructure required includes scientific expertise, research space and equipment, and secure research budgets. Scientists involved in the research enterprise typically serve the clinical mission of testing as well, the latter having priority in time and attention because of the pressing needs of patients. Commercial laboratories aligned with academic medical centers tend to be better tied to personnel involved in discovery. However, commercial laboratories are typically required to separate research effort, space, and equipment from those used to test patient samples in order to avoid the additional regulatory effort patient testing areas require for maintenance, documentation, and audit. This additional operationally mandated regulatory quality control effort is often counterproductive in a research environment. Should space and equipment be shared for research and patient testing, then there may be competition for time and access, if insufficient space and equipment capacity are encountered. Finally, research budgets may be sacrificed to the vagaries of clinical testing demands and the ebb and flow of laboratory revenues.

Outsourcing R&D, however, may also add unexpected costs from project management overhead, legal and patent fees, and royalties.[8] Dependency on outsourcing R&D risks loss of in-house expertise because of dissolution of research groups, personnel attrition, and minimization of in-house learning processes. Potential pitfalls in outsourcing include choosing a poor partner because of discordance in research or development cultures between the entities, conflicting business models, absence of transparency into partner operations, and leakage of intellectual property.

Access to patient samples is a serious challenge to commercial laboratories. Although commercial laboratories access thousands of patient samples daily, they are typically accompanied by limited clinical information, typically name, age, and *International Classification of Diseases, Tenth Revision* diagnostic code. Clinical laboratories do not usually have institutional human subjects internal review boards (IRBs), and seeking approval for research protocols and access to patient materials requires engaging an independent IRB or seeking academic or government partners who do have IRBs. Commercial laboratories do not manage patients nor follow cohorts of patients with defined disease. Hence, commercial laboratories must seek partnerships with academic or government collaborators. Defining disease groups is complicated by heterogeneity, namely variable clinical presentations for a single pathogenic pathway or variable pathogenic pathways that lead to a common clinical presentation. Selecting patients to study is often complicated by the absence of diagnostic gold standards. Verification of the utility of a new diagnostic test may require outcomes studies, usually difficult for laboratories to perform, especially for disease states that are chronic and progress over an extended period of time.

Although some neurologic diseases are relatively common, such as Alzheimer disease (AD), other conditions, such as autoimmune encephalitis, are more esoteric. For very rare diseases, identifying diagnostic biomarkers requires collaborations sufficient to collect a cohort of patients who can provide adequate phenotypic description of disease features associated with the biomarker and confirm the specificity of the biomarker for that disease. Commercial laboratories have come to heavily rely on manufacturers to perform biomarker discovery and ready-to-test reagents and assay kits. Most manufacturers, like Pharma, rely on licensing new biomarkers from university or biotechnology sources. Since the passage of the 1980 Bayh-Dole Act allowing federally funded universities and other nonprofit institutions to own intellectual property derived from federally funded research, universities have been incentivized to commercialize university-developed testing.[9] Few manufacturers maintain internal research infrastructures for discovery. Despite these challenges, several commercial clinical laboratories have found avenues to successfully bring new biomarkers to validation.

IDENTIFICATION OF NOVEL TARGET ANTIGENS

In neuroimmunology, discovery of novel biomarkers may begin with an unusual clinical presentation, but more often curiosity is raised in the laboratory by an atypical immunofluorescence pattern on brain tissue substrate, or a typical immunofluorescence pattern without identification of known autoantibodies on single analyte testing, for example, by line blots or immunofluorescence on cell substrates expressing recombinant proteins. Serum expressing these unidentified fluorescent objects, "UFOs," may be incubated with brain lysates, allowing antibody to form immune complexes with the unknown target; the immune complex is then precipitated by anti-human immunoglobulin coupled to magnetic beads, then the precipitated proteins eluted and chromatographed. Candidate proteins may then be characterized by matrix-assisted laser desorption/ionization–time of flight mass spectrometry by peptide mass fingerprinting methods.[10] The proteins may then be incorporated into prototype single-analyte assays. Clinical studies are required to confirm that the identified protein is indeed a biomarker of a given disease. In this way, several novel biomarkers have been discovered, including those associated with autoimmune cerebellar syndromes (eg, Homer protein homolog 3, inositol 1,4,5-trisphosphate receptor type 1, sodium/potassium-transporting ATPase subunit alpha-3, NCDN, Rho-associated protein kinase 2, and neurochondrin autoantibodies) and multiple sclerosis (flotillin autoantibody).[10]

Once a novel biomarker is discovered and clinically validated, a commercial laboratory must acquire or license the intellectual property in order to develop a laboratory developed test (LDT) or await a manufacturer to do so and develop the reagents or compose an assay kit that will be useable in a clinical laboratory. Attributes of an offered test the laboratory will seek include stability of supply chain, consistency of performance across manufactured lots, stability of reagents, ease of use, adaptability to automation and high-throughput testing, and cost of test performance.

The laboratory will consider cost of testing, including reagents or kit, equipment, labor, royalties, and licensing fees and weigh the costs against anticipated reimbursement. Labeling a test research use only (RUO) prejudices a test because little or no reimbursement may be expected from federal and most private insurance payers.[11] Food and Drug Administration (FDA) -approved tests are preferred because adoption of such testing often only requires the laboratory to verify that the test performs as described by the manufacturer. Although LDT assays receive comparable reimbursement to FDA-approved tests, the laboratory is required to perform a more extensive validation of the test's analytical performance, adding to development costs and time. The extent of the validation studies depends somewhat on whether the test will be qualitative, semiquantitative, or quantitative. Validation will typically include intraassay precision, interassay precision, reference interval for normality, stability, and interfering substances, but quantitative assays will also require determination of limit of detection, demonstration of linearity across an analytically measurable range, and determination of the clinically reportable range. The FDA has considered regulating LDT assays, but its current position on this is unresolved.[12–14]

High-throughput commercial laboratories with large volumes of testing also require robustness and efficiency in testing equipment platforms. Automation equipment designed for routine laboratory testing often fails when challenged in commercial laboratories by the sheer volume of tests and the duration of continuous running of the equipment. Because turnaround time is a critical parameter monitored by client hospitals and medical providers, commercial laboratories must include platform robustness in the calculation of test viability, which is true for biomarkers for common diseases as well as for those biomarkers for esoteric diseases. Esoteric test development, however, offers additional challenges. All test development requires clinically characterized analyte-positive samples in sufficient sample volume for validation studies. Esoteric diseases are esoteric. Patients with rare diseases may be difficult to find, and therefore, obtaining samples positive for novel biomarkers are also difficult. Efforts required to obtain such samples may delay development and validation pipelines. Within the neurology space, efforts to establish consortia of medical practitioners to create patient networks and pool samples in central repositories with associated clinical data have been made. One of the most successful has been the Alzheimer's Disease Neuroimaging Initiative.[15] However, similar networks in more esoteric diseases are still early in development. Lay initiated organizations, for example, the Autoimmune Encephalitis Alliance, are attracting patients and families with common interest in developing such research networks.[16]

READY OR NOT?

Before deciding to develop an assay, commercial laboratories try to anticipate market acceptance. Estimating disease incidence and prevalence is a first step, but data may vary greatly depending on the disease and available sources. The availability of a novel therapeutic often drives the need for specific diagnostic tests to aid in therapy selection. When guidelines are available, market estimates may be inferred by predicted patient populations. Similarly, when an analyte is designated a companion or complementary diagnostic test for an accepted or newly approved therapy, market size can be estimated on prior accumulated or anticipated drug usage data, respectively. For esoteric diseases, the data may not exist. Common diseases have often been extensively studied. Professional society guidelines may help in these instances, but few guidelines for testing exist for esoteric tests, and fewer exist still for novel biomarkers new to medical practice. Assays to detect disease-specific biomarkers with increased seropositivity rates would be easier for commercial laboratories to adopt compared with idiopathic disorders with unclear prevalence and limited seropositivity rates; guidelines effecting diagnostic criteria can alter this calculus.[17] However, even when a newly introduced biomarker assay meets a medical need, adoption may be slow, requiring education of practitioners as to its nature and role in disease diagnosis or management. For example, the prevalence of neuromyelitis optica spectrum disorder (NMOSD) is approximately 1 to 10 per 100,000 individuals, globally.[18] Approximately 73% to 90% of diagnosed NMOSD patients have Aquaporin-4 antibodies.[19] Because the association of Aquaporin-4 antibodies met the pressing need for a biomarker to assist in diagnosis of a challenging idiopathic disease and its differentiation from multiple sclerosis, development of guidelines was accelerated and aided physician education.[19,20] Commercial laboratories participate in medical education, but investment in continuing medical education is typically modest compared with Pharma.

Another concern is that there are an increasing number of biomarkers being identified through preclinical research, but with limited known clinical utility, thereby impeding market approval.[21] These tests continue to be offered by the manufacturer only as RUO assays until the required intended use of the biomarker is accepted by clinical communities. Clinical utility of a biomarker will ultimately depend on validated measurements that are accurately reproduced across clinical settings and institutions.[22] Therefore, to move an RUO marker from research to clinical utility requires multidisciplinary collaborations between academic institutions and in vitro diagnostic companies, before being adopted by commercial laboratories. The lack of disease-specific biomarkers is one of the major challenges to creating "the right biomarker, the right drug, for the right patient."[21,22]

Autoimmune neurologic disorders are complex diseases that often require collaboration among multiple medical disciplines for effective diagnosis and treatment. Because of a lack of a uniform and standardized diagnostic algorithm adopted by a consensus in the clinical community, drafting of testing algorithms and strategies fall in the hands of laboratory directors, in turn making the results laboratory dependent.[23–25] In addition, analysis of autoimmune neurology test results requires intensive training of technicians in fluorescence pattern recognition often resulting in outcomes that are somewhat subjective and reader specific. In addition, lack of uniform cutoff values, certified reference materials (CRM), restricted regulatory approval, lack of validation samples, intensive validation measures, and low reimbursements values, all pose additional challenges to commercial laboratories contemplating bringing autoimmune neurology testing onboard.

Commercial laboratories may also be reluctant to bring in assays for neurologic disorders, despite the disorder having known prevalence and increased mortalities, because they lack diagnostic guidelines and regulatory approvals. Neurodegenerative disorders, including AD, fall into this category of disorders that lack highly disease-correlated biomarkers that can provide reliable outcomes, despite being prevalent diseases. Neurodegeneration is the underlying mechanism behind many diseases, such as AD, Parkinson disease, and motor neuron diseases, and is often difficult to diagnose using a single assay. Despite decades of research in this field, there has been no single biomarker that can facilitate robust prospective prediction of neurodegenerative diseases or aid in selection of appropriate therapeutic target.[26]

AD is the most common cause of dementia in the elderly and is observed in 70% of dementia cases.[27] AD is considered the sixth leading cause of death in the United States with 15% of Americans over age 60 years having prodromal AD and close to 40% having preclinical AD.[28] Overall, 5.8 million Americans suffer from AD, and it is expected to increase to approximately 13 million by 2050.[27] Despite these statistics and persistent efforts by investigators, identifying clinically relevant biomarkers has proven a highly challenging task in neurodegenerative diseases, including AD. In 2011, the National Institute on Aging and the Alzheimer Association Workgroup revised the diagnostic guidelines for AD after 27 years and recognized the potential use of biomarkers to diagnose AD.[29] Abnormal levels of biomarkers, including amyloid and tau, are noticeable approximately 10 to 20 years before the onset of clinical symptoms. However, incorporation of such biomarkers in routine clinical practice is modest compared with preclinical research.[29] In recent years, extensive studies were conducted to further understand the relationship of amyloid and tau biomarkers to onset of symptoms and correlation with postmortem studies. Excellent correlations are observed between challenging sample matrix (CSF) beta-amyloid 42/40 ratio values and ^{18}F-flutemetamol-labeled PET imaging results in AD patients. However, high levels of discordance are noted in cognitively healthy and memory complaint subjects.[30,31] Lack of knowledge regarding such discordance and in turn pathophysiologic changes in neurodegeneration has impaired development of ideal candidate diagnostic and prognostic biomarkers in AD.

In addition to measuring protein biomarkers, such as amyloid and tau in the CSF, there have been an increasing number of biomarkers identified through preclinical research, but with limited clinical utility. Such research markers may not be fit for clinical trial or clinical practice because of lack of robust and reliable diagnostic assays. Furthermore, studies have shown high variability in measuring biomarker concentrations in equivalent sample sets evaluated in different laboratories, despite using the same methodology. Such large variabilities have hindered establishment of global cutoff values for AD biomarkers and are largely due to variations in preanalytical procedures (sample collection and handling), analytical procedures, and differences in production of biomarker tests.[32] The 2011 guidelines dictated the need to have biomarkers tests that have standardized, reliable, and reproducible diagnostic caliber readouts.[29] Lack of CRM could result in systemic bias of measured biomarker concentrations across different assays. In 2017, the first CRM was developed for measuring beta-amyloid 42, and CRM for measuring other AD biomarkers are currently under development.[33] Lack of standardized test systems in neurodegeneration has made biomarker outcomes vendor dependent, making it difficult for commercial laboratories to choose the accurate test method for identifying such conditions. In addition, to date, there is no regulatory approval for neurodegenerative biomarkers in the United States forcing the laboratories to offer these tests only as LDTs. Altogether, lack of FDA-recognized intended use or clinical utility of the biomarker, absence of professional society guidelines and regulatory approval, CSF, increased level of validation and qualification for offering the tests as LDT, and lower reimbursements rates have made it extremely difficult for commercial laboratories to adopt diagnostic tests for neurodegenerative conditions.

MORE IS LESS, LESS IS MORE

Commercial laboratories depend on economy of scale to keep internal costs low. Client hospitals, provider systems, and payers depend on competition to drive their costs lower. The retail price of testing does not often reflect negotiated contract pricing because testing volume can reduce negotiated costs to clients. Often the price of common laboratory tests gradually declines over time as competition and gradual improvements in testing decrease internal costs for laboratories that may be passed on to clients. For rare disease biomarkers, however, it is often difficult to achieve economy of scale. In addition, the methodology may inherently be costlier. Manufacturers may have added costs from licensing royalties, small production runs because of limited product movement and short shelf life, and the effort required to manufacture unusual recombinant proteins. In the commercial laboratory, test performance may be more labor intensive and require highly trained staff. For example, detection of auto-antibodies to brain begins with screening patient serum or CSF on multiple neurologic tissues in immunofluorescent assays.[23] Although automated systems exist for slide preparation and image acquisition, testing still requires a highly trained technologist to review images and interpret patterns of tissue staining.[34] Similarly, trained technologists are required for interpretation of analyte-specific recombinant cell-based immunofluorescence assays.[34,35] The testing algorithms are complex because a given clinical presentation may be caused by several different autoantibodies, a given auto-antibody may cause several different diseases, tissue immunofluorescence staining patterns may be subtle, and different patterns overlap.[34,36] Training requires dedicated time that removes technologists from the routine work flow and productivity during their training time. The required time for testing and test interpretation, complexity, and labor intensity in these esoteric tests makes them costly. However, laboratory test cost and the correct diagnosis it can afford need to be measured, for example, in auto-immune encephalitis cases, which often require an intensive care unit admission, against the cost of prolonged hospitalization and the cost to the hospital system, and more importantly to the patient, of worsening morbidity, or even death.[37] The importance of an early and correct diagnosis in neurologic disease, particularly when intervention can minimize damage and save lives, is immeasurable.

DISCLOSURE

I. Venkataraman is employed by EUROIMMUN US; S.J. Naides is employed by EURO-IMMUN US; was formerly employed by Quest Diagnostics, Inc.

REFERENCES

1. Ehrmeyer SS, Laessig RH. Has compliance with CLIA requirements really improved quality in US clinical laboratories? Clin Chim Acta 2004;346:37–43.
2. Hess N. CLIA and regulatory readiness: how can your lab always be ready? MLO Med Lab Obs 2016;48:38, 40, 42 passim.
3. Hamlin W. Proficiency testing as a regulatory device: a CAP perspective. Clin Chem 1992;38(7):1234–50.
4. Lawson NS. Quality assurance programs in the United States. Ann Ist Super Sanita 1995;31(1):21–35.
5. Buvailo A. Pharma R&D outsourcing is on the rise. 2020. Available at: https://www.biopharmatrend.com/post/30-pharma-rd-outsourcing-is-on-the-rise/. Accessed January 13, 2020.
6. Schuhmacher A, Trill H, Gassmann O. Models for open innovation in the pharmaceutical industry. Drug Discov Today 2013;18:1133–7.
7. "The CRO Market" Archived 2013-07-03 at the Wayback Machine, Association of Clinical Research Organizations. Available at: https://web.archive.org/web/20100311082536/http://www.acrohealth.org/cro-market.php. Aaccessed April 7, 2010.

8. Baier E, Rammer C, Schuber T. The impact on innovation off-shoring on organizational adaptability, ZEW Discussion Papers, No. 13-109, Zentrum für Europäische Wirtschaftsforschung (ZEW), Mannheim. 2013. Available at: http://nbn-resolving.de/urn:nbn:de:bsz:180-madoc-353018. Accessed June 21, 2020.

9. Drozdoff V, Fairbairn D. Licensing biotech intellectual property in university–industry partnerships. Cold Spring Harb Perspect Med 2015;5:a021014.

10. Scharf M, Miske R, Kade S, et al. A spectrum of neural autoantigens, newly identified by histo-immunoprecipitation, mass spectrometry, and recombinant cell-based indirect immunofluorescence. Front Immunol 2018;9:1447.

11. Takemura Y, Beck JR. The effects of a fixed-fee reimbursement system introduced by the federal government on laboratory testing in the United States. Rinsho Byori 1999;47(1):1–10.

12. Thompson BM, Scott BI, Boiani JA. Understanding the Food and Drug Administration's jurisdiction over laboratory-developed tests and divisions between food, drug, and cosmetic act-regulated and clinical laboratory improvement amendments of 1988-regulated activities. Clin Lab Med 2016;36(3):575–85.

13. Genzen JR, Mohlman JS, Lynch JL, et al. Laboratory-developed tests: a legislative and regulatory review. Clin Chem 2017;63(10):1575–84.

14. Genzen JR. Regulation of laboratory-developed tests. Am J Clin Pathol 2019; 152(2):122–31.

15. Weiner MW, Veitch DP, Aisen PS, et al. Recent publications from the Alzheimer's Disease Neuroimaging Initiative: reviewing progress toward improved AD clinical trials. Alzheimers Dement 2017;13(4):e1–85.

16. Available at: https://aealliance.org/. Accessed May 20, 2020.

17. Hamid SH, Elsone L, Mutch K, et al. The impact of 2015 neuromyelitis optica spectrum disorders criteria on diagnostic rates. Mult Scler 2017;23(2):228–33.

18. Available at: https://rarediseases.org/rare-diseases/neuromyelitis-optica/. Accessed May 20, 2020.

19. Whittam D, Wilson M, Hamid S, et al. What's new in neuromyelitis optica? A short review for the clinical neurologist. J Neurol 2017;264:2330–44.

20. Wingerchuk DM, Banwell B, Bennett JL, et al. International consensus diagnostic criteria for neuromyelitis optica spectrum disorders. Neurology 2015;85(2): 177–89.

21. Wang X, Ward PA. Opportunities and challenges of disease biomarkers: a new section in the journal of translational medicine. J Transl Med 2012;10:220.

22. Lucs A, Saltman B, Chung CH, et al. Opportunities and challenges facing biomarker development for personalized head and neck cancer treatment. Head Neck 2013;35(2):294–306.

23. Graus F, Delattre JY, Antoine JC, et al. Recommended diagnostic criteria for paraneoplastic neurological syndromes. J Neurol Neurosurg Psychiatry 2004;75(8): 1135–40.

24. Graus F, Titulaer MJ, Balu R, et al. A clinical approach to diagnosis of autoimmune encephalitis. Lancet Neurol 2016;15(4):391–404.

25. Höftberger R. Neuroimmunology: an expanding frontier in autoimmunity. Front Immunol 2015;6:206.

26. Hu CJ, Octave JN. Editorial: risk factors and outcome predicating biomarker of neurodegenerative diseases. Front Neurol 2019;10:45.

27. Alzheimer's disease facts and figures. Available at: https://www.alz.org/media/documents/alzheimers-facts-and-figures-2019-r.pdf. Accessed May 25, 2020.

28. Mar J, Soto-Gordoa M, Arrospide A, et al. Fitting the epidemiology and neuropathology of the early stages of Alzheimer's disease to prevent dementia. Alzheimers Res Ther 2015;7(1):2.
29. Jack CR Jr, Albert MS, Knopman DS, et al. Introduction to the recommendations from the National Institute on Aging-Alzheimer's Association workgroups on diagnostic guidelines for Alzheimer's disease. Alzheimers Dement 2011;7(3):257–62.
30. Leuzy A, Chiotis K, Hasselbalch SG, et al. Pittsburgh compound B imaging and cerebrospinal fluid amyloid-β in a multicentre European Memory Clinic Study. Brain 2016;139(Pt 9):2540–53.
31. Palmqvist S, Mattsson N, Hansson O, Alzheimer's Disease Neuroimaging Initiative. Cerebrospinal fluid analysis detects cerebral amyloid-β accumulation earlier than positron emission tomography. Brain 2016;139(Pt 4):1226–36.
32. Bjerke M, Andreasson U, Kuhlmann J, et al. Assessing the commutability of reference material formats for the harmonization of amyloid-β measurements. Clin Chem Lab Med 2016;54(7):1177–91.
33. Kuhlmann J, Boulo S, Andreasson U, et al. Certification REPORT: the certification of amyloid β1-42 in CSF in ERM®-DA480/IFCC, ERM®-DA481/IFCC and ERM®-DA482/IFCC: European Commission. 2017. Available at: https://ec.europa.eu/jrc/en/publication/eur-scientific-andtechnical- research-reports/certification-report-certification-amyloid- 1-42-csf-erm-da480ifcc-erm-da481ifcc-and-erm. Accessed May 20, 2020.
34. Naides SJ. The role of the laboratory in the expanding field of neuroimmunology: autoantibodies to neural targets. J Immunol Methods 2018;463:1–20.
35. Honorat JA, Komorowski L, Josephs KA, et al. IgLON5 antibody: neurological accompaniments and outcomes in 20 patients. Neurol Neuroimmunol Neuroinflamm 2017;4(5):e385.
36. Darnell RB, Posner JB. Paraneoplastic syndromes. Oxford (England): Oxford University Press; 2011.
37. Cohen J, Sotoca J, Gandhi S, et al. Autoimmune encephalitis: a costly condition. Neurology 2019;92:e964–72.

Something's Lost and Something's Gained
Seeing Reference Laboratory Quality from Both Sides, Now

Yael K. Heher, MD, MPH, FRCP(C)*

KEYWORDS

- Patient safety • Reference laboratory • Testing • Quality assurance
- Quality improvement • Test cycle • Laboratory management

KEY POINTS

- Health care reimbursement and regulatory changes along with an increase in the number and complexity of available tests have led many hospital and practice-based laboratories and physicians to embrace the use of reference laboratories to meet their clinical needs at a lower cost and burden.
- The concept of testing neutrality, introduced by Clinical Laboratory Improvement Amendments (CLIA) 1988, states that the responsibility for testing quality lies with the referring provider group or laboratory. Outsourcing a laboratory test does not alter this responsibility.
- Safety vulnerabilities exist in all phases of laboratory testing, but particularly problematic for tests sent to reference laboratories are the pre-analytic and post-analytic phases involving test ordering, decision support, and test result interface.
- Integration of the reference laboratory information system with the local laboratory information system and the electronic health record is critical to reduce error.
- Oversight of clinical reference laboratory performance is complex and fragmented. Leaders must exert deliberate collaborative ownership of the full test cycle to address gaps in safety and quality.

THE ALLURE OF REFERENCE LABORATORIES

Reference laboratories are laboratories typically located in separate geographic locations that receive specimens called "send-outs" from a "referring" laboratory, and perform one or more tests on such specimens. Reference laboratory testing offers

---

* Department of Pathology and Laboratory Medicine, Quality and Patient Safety, Beth Israel Deaconess Medical Center, 330 Brookline Avenue, FN201 Boston, MA 02215, USA
E-mail address: ykheher@bidmc.harvard.edu
Twitter: @yaelheher (Y.K.H.)

Clin Lab Med 40 (2020) 341–356
https://doi.org/10.1016/j.cll.2020.05.007
0272-2712/20/© 2020 Elsevier Inc. All rights reserved.
labmed.theclinics.com

an appealing and necessary alternative to on-site testing for referring laboratories of all types and sizes. Reference laboratories have the ability to perform esoteric, challenging, and varied testing at a high volume and quality and at a relatively low cost. For rare tests, reference laboratories may also provide specialized consultative assistance. Hospitals and other providers considering the use of reference laboratories for particular tests face a classic "make or buy" decision. Considerations include cost, in-house availability of required expertise and instrumentation, and availability of technologists and staff to ensure service needs.[1]

Increasing regulatory burdens, decreasing reimbursements, increased number and complexity of available tests, and the notion of laboratory services as a commodity have put immense pressure on laboratories everywhere.[2–7] Reference laboratories address increasing demands from patients and families for result portals and commercial-level customer service. Larger reference laboratories compete for business with direct to consumer marketing campaigns highlighting these services. To encourage referring laboratories, hospitals, or ordering providers to enter into service contracts, reference laboratories may provide on-site phlebotomy and courier services. For larger customers, reference laboratories may provide additional on-site employees to log in and triage specimens. Quest Diagnostics Laboratories, for example, has more than 2250 "patient service centers" and provides phlebotomy and test intake in more than 4000 additional locations.[8] In addition to private large laboratory groups, academic medical center laboratories or main hospital laboratories that are part of a large system may act as reference laboratories for their partners and affiliates. The Beth Israel Deaconess Medical Center Division of Laboratory Medicine performs 6 to 7 million tests per year; 200,000 (3%) of these are send-out tests, which cost the pathology department in excess of $4 million per year. Some of these costs are recovered from the patients' insurance providers, but in certain situations, for testing performed on inpatients, no reimbursement is available, and depending on payor mix, cost may exceed reimbursement in other cases. Over the past 2 decades, division of laboratory medicine reference laboratory testing volume at our institution has increased 10-fold, from 20 to 25,000 to 200 to 250,000 tests per year (Beth Israel Deaconess Medical Center, unpublished data).

RESPONSIBILITY FOR QUALITY

The growth of reference laboratories raises important questions regarding regulation, oversight, and responsibility for quality and safety. The Clinical Laboratory Improvement Amendments of 1988 (CLIA '88) introduced the concept of "Testing Site Neutrality," which requires that a referring laboratory ensure the quality of laboratory testing irrespective of where testing is performed.[9,10] CLIA '88 mandates that the main laboratory be responsible for integration with quality control and quality assurance, regulatory requirements and certification, and training and education.[2,10] Referring laboratory leadership must therefore be intimately acquainted with reference laboratory processes and cognizant of safety risks.

Regulation and interest in the accuracy of diagnostic testing extend well beyond CLIA. The National Academy of Medicine's 2015 follow-up report to "To Err is Human" included the failure to correctly communicate results in its definition of "diagnostic error."[11] The Society to Improve Diagnosis, the Agency for Healthcare Research and Quality, and the Centers for Medicare and Medicaid Services have all focused funding, regulatory, and legislative efforts on reducing diagnostic error.[12–17]

Implications of Testing Site Neutrality on Laboratory Quality Programs

Most referring laboratories take basic steps to comply with CLIA '88. The referring laboratory's Standard Operating Procedures will state that it has verified the reference laboratory's CLIA license, and that it monitors agreed-on quality metrics typically centered around billing, cost, and turnaround time (TAT). These metrics are monitored at some regular interval and are often not revisited over the life cycle of the service contract.

In reality, effective monitoring of send-out laboratory quality requires a much more comprehensive approach. Even a well-known and simple metric like TAT can be inaccurate and misleading in the world of send-outs. The reference laboratory may monitor TAT from their own accessioning to resulting, while the referring laboratory may monitor the pre-analytic time to sending out the specimen, or may not. Often neither laboratory monitors transport time or post-analytic delays in reporting the result. The true TAT from the perspective of the patient or ordering provider "client" is never captured. Interface issues affecting formatting and result reporting and interpretation can have a major impact on patient safety, can make the process seem incomplete and fragmented for ordering providers, and are almost never routinely monitored or reported. When the responsibility for measuring process and outcomes measures falls between reference and referring laboratories, meaningful quality data are in short supply.

SAFETY RISK IN ALL PHASES OF THE TEST CYCLE

Both referring and reference laboratories focus heavily on quality control and proficiency of their own analytical testing with considerable success. But a more expansive definition of quality goes beyond analysis to include all phases of the test cycle, while accounting for the impact on patient outcomes.[2,6,18–25] Novel and unexpected quality and safety problems arise all along the test cycle when referring laboratories send a specimen to a reference laboratory. Frequent setbacks in the pre-analytic phase include difficulties with specimen transport and integrity, duplicate accessioning, and login delays. In the post-analytic phase, failures in the communication of results are common and often result from problems with the interface of separate information systems. Even the analytical phase is not immune, as errors can occur if the reference laboratory misses important clinical data, such as interfering medications or preexisting antibodies. Without access to the patient's electronic health record (EHR), clinical context, and local medical director review, reference laboratories may be unable to correctly interpret unusual test results. Differentiating between analytical error and true physiologic conditions may be impossible, creating additional patient safety risk.

Like a fly ball falling between 2 outfielders, errors in the pre- and post-analytic phases are particularly problematic when neither the referring nor the reference laboratory take ownership. The baseline pre- and post-analytic risks are doubled when referring and reference laboratories interact, and then are amplified by the new risks related to information technology (IT) interface and communication. Quality and patient safety considerations for all phases of laboratory testing are reviewed in **Fig. 1**.

USING CHECKLISTS AND QUALITY METRICS TO OPTIMIZE SAFETY IN REFERENCE LABORATORY TESTING

Successful management of the risks associated with reference laboratories requires deliberate implementation and assessment of processes using validated quality and safety tools. Reference laboratory quality metrics must be defined, agreed on by diverse stakeholders, incorporated into contracts, and regularly monitored. A dashboard can be a useful tool for real-time measurement and reporting of standardized

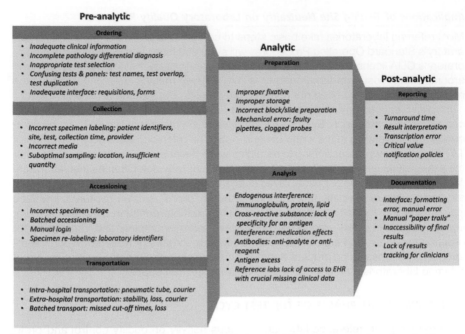

Pre-analytic

Ordering
- *Inadequate clinical information*
- *Incomplete pathology differential diagnosis*
- *Inappropriate test selection*
- *Confusing tests & panels: test names, test overlap, test duplication*
- *Inadequate interface: requisitions, forms*

Collection
- *Incorrect specimen labeling: patient identifiers, site, test, collection time, provider*
- *Incorrect media*
- *Suboptimal sampling: location, insufficient quantity*

Accessioning
- *Incorrect specimen triage*
- *Batched accessioning*
- *Manual login*
- *Specimen re-labeling: laboratory identifiers*

Transportation
- *Intra-hospital transportation: pneumatic tube, courier*
- *Extra-hospital transportation: stability, loss, courier*
- *Batched transport: missed cut-off times, loss*

Analytic

Preparation
- *Improper fixative*
- *Improper storage*
- *Incorrect block/slide preparation*
- *Mechanical error: faulty pipettes, clogged probes*

Analysis
- *Endogenous interference: immunoglobulin, protein, lipid*
- *Cross-reactive substance: lack of specificity for an antigen*
- *Interference: medication effects*
- *Antibodies: anti-analyte or anti-reagent*
- *Antigen excess*
- *Reference labs lack of access to EHR with crucial missing clinical data*

Post-analytic

Reporting
- *Turnaround time*
- *Result interpretation*
- *Transcription error*
- *Critical value notification policies*

Documentation
- *Interface: formatting error, manual error*
- *Manual "paper trails"*
- *Inaccessibility of final results*
- *Lack of results tracking for clinicians*

Fig. 1. Quality and safety considerations in all phases of the reference laboratory testing cycle. Major and frequently overlooked risk exists in pre-analytic and post-analytic phases of the test cycle.

quality data by using visual cues, run charts, and statistical process control.[23,26–29] **Table 1** lists potential quality metrics to consider when monitoring reference laboratory performance and corresponding examples of compliance.

Safety checklists can be effective tools to ensure reliability of complex processes, such as referring-reference laboratory relationships.[30–34] **Table 2** is a proposed checklist and worksheet for use by referring laboratories to improve the management of reference laboratory testing. The checklist specifies task ownership, relevant notes, and target dates, while using color cues to indicate task completion.

THE INESTIMABLE VALUE OF CLINICAL FEEDBACK

Sophisticated and well-established laboratory quality programs are proactive and integrate the tools described previously. However, in the complex business of caring for patients, unexpected problems inevitably arise, thus laboratory leaders must have a mechanism for obtaining critical feedback retrospectively from ordering providers and patients. A laboratory-centric, reactive stance is less effective at preventing harm than one that embraces the preferences of treating clinicians, patients, and families.[35–39] **Table 3** lists common complaints from treating neurologists, as an example, and other ordering providers about reference laboratory testing and proposed solutions.

SPECIAL SITUATIONS IN REFERENCE LABORATORY TESTING

Referring laboratory leaders face additional quality and safety challenges when approving a new test for outsourcing, when converting an existing test to a send-out, or when bringing a send-out test in-house. When considering offering a new

Table 1	
Proposed quality metrics to be monitored regarding reference laboratory testing and sample evidence of compliance	
Quality Metric	**Evidence of Compliance**
Laboratory licensure, accreditation, certification	Current CLIA certificates, Joint Commission or College of American Pathologists accreditation, FDA approval
Ordering provider satisfaction	TAT, test frequency, qualitative survey feedback data from ordering providers
Client services support and responsiveness	Number of errors addressed promptly and thoroughly, TAT for error responses
Lost or compromised specimens	Error rate, nature of error: handoff, interface, clerical, analytical, interpretative
"Carrots and sticks"	Consider specific performance metrics and targets that would result in financial incentives or penalties

These should be adapted to referring laboratories' specific vulnerabilities and needs.

Abbreviations: CLIA, Clinical Laboratory Improvement Amendment 1988; FDA, US Food and Drug Administration; TAT, turnaround time.

test offered by a reference laboratory, laboratory leaders must assess both the clinical and research relevance of the test and the associated revenue streams. For existing tests that are being considered for outsourcing, changes to the ordering process, TAT, and the reporting of results must be discussed in detail. For tests that may be candidates to be brought in-house, when ordering volume reaches a certain threshold, for example, leaders must confirm that appropriate expertise, personnel, and testing infrastructure are available. A new medical director with specialized skills, or new instrumentation or laboratory space may be required for successful transition. Laboratory leaders should consider what redundancy is required for equipment and personnel, and ensure that a backup system or process is available for time-sensitive, critical tests. In all cases, the laboratory leaders should assemble a multidisciplinary group of requesting clinicians, laboratorians, administrators, contractors, and regulators to review and create consensus over each proposal. This group should reassemble after implementation to revisit laboratory testing processes, to audit for pre-analytic and post-analytic error, and seek ordering provider feedback to allow for continuous improvement. The reference laboratory new test planning cycle is reviewed in **Fig. 2**.

THE CRITICAL ROLE OF HEALTH INFORMATION TECHNOLOGY

Although IT system interoperability is critical to all clinical pathology testing, the risks of poor interoperability are multiplied, amplified, and made more complex by the introduction of reference laboratories. Thoughtful design and integration of laboratory information systems, provider ordering systems, and the EHR between referring and reference laboratory providers remains the single most important factor in pre-analytic and post-analytic quality and safety. **Fig. 3** illustrates suboptimal (left) and optimal (right) states of IT integration in reference laboratory testing.

Safety risks exist in nearly every aspect of IT integration.[40–42] Regulators and policy makers at the highest levels have targeted this immense risk relatively unsuccessfully.[43] Even the formatting of an abnormal result, which may seem like a simple task appropriate for a junior programmer, can have significant impact on how ordering providers respond to the result.[44] Examples from my institution are in **Fig. 4**. If

Table 2
Reference laboratory testing implementation safety checklist

Checklist Task	Owner(s) Name, Role (Example)	Notes	Complete? Y/N	Target Date
Have the appropriate treating clinical teams been involved in test selection?	Neurology Chief	Needs input from inpatient leaders and outpatient affiliates	Y	
Will the test impact clinical care and/or discovery?	Chiefs of Neurology, Director of Neuroscience research	Upload data and articles to request package	Y	
Has the Pathology Service Committee reviewed?	Pathology Services Committee Chair and multidisciplinary members	Confirm with Lab Medicine Chief before approval	Y	
Has the billing process been planned and approved?	Chief Administrative Officer, Pathology and hospital billing leadership	Confirm process with payors, confirm process with vendors	N	
Has the IT process been planned with the reference laboratory?	Reference laboratory leadership, collaborative	Who will own integration? What metrics will be monitored to determine quality of the interface?	N	
Has the IT process been planned with the referring laboratory?	Laboratory information systems leadership, collaborative	Resolve interface formatting	N	
Has the IT process been planned with the hospital or system electronic health record team?	Electronic health record leadership, collaborative	Will results appear under the typical laboratory results tab? Under a separate tab?	N	
How will consent requirements be handled?	Collaborative leadership	What are the legal requirements of the referring and reference laboratories?	Y	
Has the testing been adequately piloted before go-live?	Collaborative IT leadership	Consider rare scenarios	N	
Have treating clinicians/customers been consulted after go-live on satisfaction and functionality?	Collaborative laboratory, clinical leadership	Is there a clear mechanism for users to report errors and issues?	N	
Have laboratory and clinical leadership selected meaningful quality metrics to monitor?	Collaborative, reference, and main laboratory, treating clinical leadership	Parse out pre- and post-analytic TAT from reference laboratory TAT. Ensure mechanism to report and monitor formatting errors affecting safety. Monitor utilization and overlap of test panels?	Y	

What is the ownership and process for critical value (CV) reporting?	Collaborative, reference and main laboratory, treating clinical leadership	Does the reference laboratory CV list match the referring laboratories'? Will some CVs be held during non-business hours? Is the CV list approved by treating clinical leadership? Who will be responsible for contacting ordering providers?	Y
Have changes been made to the process based on quality performance and user feedback?	All stakeholders	Revisit ordering, resulting, and testing based on performance and feedback	N
Have all ordering and process changes been communicated clearly to ordering providers and referring laboratories?	Main laboratory leadership	Users need to know about TAT, testing schedules, pertinent cost or documentation requirements, and whom to contact in the laboratory with questions or issues	Y

Laboratory leaders of referring laboratories should strongly consider using the checklist as a project management dashboard and tool, color coding cells to indicate progress, and clearly defining process step ownership and target dates. In this example, red indicates incomplete tasks, whereas green indicates completed ones.

Abbreviations: CV, critical value; IT, information technology; TAT, turnaround time.

Table 3
Common complaints from treating clinicians on send-out testing and corresponding systems-based proposed solutions

Complaint Category	Complaint Quote	Proposed Systems Solution(s)
Specimen ordering and procurement	"There is no prompt for providers/phlebotomists to draw the right quantity in the right tube—frontline clinicians do not have time to look up the lab manual for every test!" "By the time the lab notifies us of an issue, the patient has to be redrawn/return—in the case of CSF this is a major problem" "I have no idea when tests are run, my patient went for a draw and then [his] specimen was rejected because testing is only performed on certain days and times and the specimen was no longer useable"	Prompts in the ordering system and hard stops on controlling specimen factors such as transport medium, volume, testing timing and frequency Example of hard stop: the specimen bar code will not let you print a label for a test that is not being performed within a certain time frame, specimen tubes can be pre-marked with volume cutoffs necessary for specific tests, and so forth
Test documentation	"I have to fill out one form for the main lab. Then I have to fill out another for the reference lab. I have to complete consent forms with the patient. I have to sign release and request forms. About a third of the time, testing is held up because of some error with documentation. Can't this be simplified?"	Streamline and consolidate referring and reference lab documentation program requirements to simplify clinical test ordering Consider sharing the documentation burden between clinical and laboratory staff as permitted by regulatory standards
Test utilization	"The internal medicine team will order every possible neurology test on a new patient with dementia before consulting neurology. The results are not useful or indicated, typically normal, and bias the lab into thinking the results are not important or urgent. Then when the consulting specialists really do need the test we can't get it done promptly."	Consider restrictions on what types of providers can order esoteric tests without special permission Consider testing algorithms, decision support for common diagnostic dilemmas
Specimen processing	"I don't even know which tests are send-outs and which are done in-house—how can I tell how fast they will be resulted?"	Note test type and TAT expectation at ordering phase to manage expectations and assist with clinical planning

Category	Quote	Recommendation
Specimen status	"When a test says 'pending' in the EHR for weeks on end, I have no idea if everything is okay and it's in progress, or if it's lost, misprocessed, or was never sent" "The EHR says SEE COMMENT but there is no comment and when I call the lab they say it hasn't been sent out yet"	Process tracking updates interfaced with EHR visible to treating clinician: bidirectional interface
TAT	"By the time the result is back it's no longer clinically relevant—the patient is critically ill and toxic and/or we can't tell if they are noncompliant with medications."	Input from treating clinicians, reference laboratory operations
Test tracking	"When patients are recently discharged, we have no way of tracking results but manual note taking and clinic follow-up because patients fall between inpatients and outpatient test tracking mechanisms."	Create safe process for result tracking of recently discharged patients
Test interpretation	"I can't tell where the actual result is on the reference lab report—the formatting changes all the time and is impossible to read." "The reference ranges change from lab to lab and then I can't tell if my patient's result is normal or abnormal."	Clear, thoughtful programming of interface format to optimize result interpretation that is, "do not bury the lead" Abnormal results need to be formatted (bold, asterisk) and reference ranges clearly noted Reference ranges should be changed only if absolutely necessary and ordering providers must be notified of changes
Financial considerations	"I have no idea what the fees are for testing. My patients can be direct billed, or reimbursement can be rejected by their insurance at great cost to them, and they are furious with me. I don't know how to manage this and I feel terrible about it." "I've ordered tests on inpatients and they are held, unbeknownst to be, until discharge because of billing optimization."	Transparency around billing process and reimbursement at the time of ordering Transparency around differences between inpatient and ambulatory care

Abbreviations: CSF, cerebrospinal fluid; EHR, electronic health record; TAT, turnaround time.

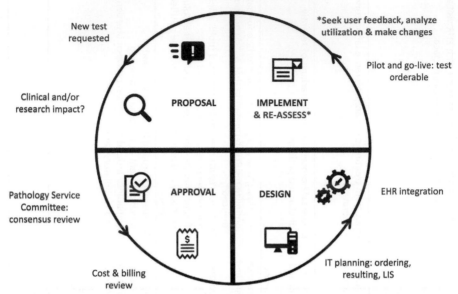

Fig. 2. The reference laboratory new test planning cycle. A frequently forgotten step is re-assessment and quality measurement of full test cycle performance post-implementation, taking into consideration feedback from laboratorians, technicians, and ordering providers.

reference laboratory systems are not fully integrated with the referring laboratory EHR, laboratory results may be faxed, mailed, or manually transcribed into the EHR, a primitive approach bedeviled by human error. Clinicians may have difficulty finding results that do not appear in the usual EHR location, only to learn that results from a particular reference laboratory appear as a scanned document elsewhere in the medical record. If the send-out test is not included in the results tracking system, the clinician may assume the test was never resulted or was not sent, and the laboratory will have no confirmation that the result was seen and acted on. Poor integration into the tracking system may contribute to frustration or alarm fatigue for providers forced to

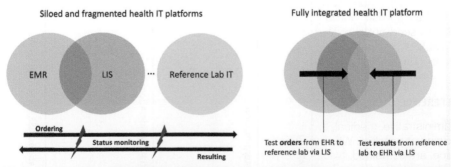

Fig. 3. Considerations in health record and laboratory information system interfacing. Functional, fully integrated IT platforms are critical to quality and patient safety. EMR, electronic medical record; LIS, laboratory information system.

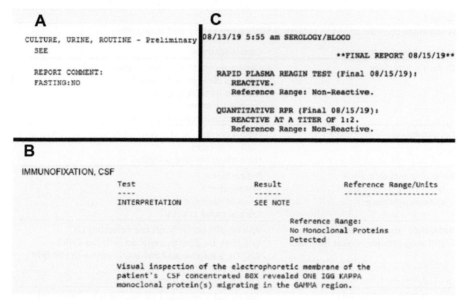

Fig. 4. Examples of patient safety vulnerabilities due to IT shortcomings in reference laboratory information systems report interface. (*A*) Report references a preliminary result, but none is available. There is a note to see report comment but no hyperlink embedded to access the comment. (*B*) This infectious disease result was missed by the clinical team due to misalignment. Despite capitalization of the actual result, a busy treating clinician scanning for test results read "Non-Reactive" as the actual result because of formatting. (*C*) The treating clinical team missed this cerebrospinal fluid (CSF) immunofixation result due to laboratory interface formatting. The result appears to be "No Monoclonal Proteins Detected," actually under "Reference Range," but on closer inspection, the true result of "IgG (IGG) kappa monoclonal protein" is hidden in a paragraph that appears from formatting more like a note regarding laboratory regulations. RPR, rapid plasma reagent.

acknowledge large volumes of normal results, or asked to acknowledge the same result that is presented repeatedly. Some institutions will maintain excellent IT communication with larger reference laboratories but not others, an inconsistency that again complicates the delivery of results. Inadequate integration of security mechanisms can create extraordinary inefficiency for staff: at my institution, send-out laboratory coordinators must key in their passwords 500 to 600 times each day to obtain and then publish individual results from reference laboratories (unpublished data, BIDMC send-out coordinator).

Table 4 lists general IT considerations in the area of reference laboratory patient safety. **Table 5** lists models of result interface in send-out testing and associated risks.

REFERENCE LABORATORY TESTING GOVERNANCE AND OVERSIGHT

Administrative, medical, and technical leadership of laboratories is intricate and challenging at baseline. When the dynamics by 2 laboratories, the referring and the reference, are combined, twice the burden and risk can result.

Thoughtful governance and reporting structures are vital. Reference laboratory testing tends to be overseen by referring laboratory medical directors in the area of testing. However, busy clinical directors and technologists may not prioritize the

Table 4
IT interface considerations in reference laboratory safety and integration

IT Integration Category	Considerations
Ordering interface	Orders direct to reference laboratory? Options clear in test menu? Overlap of testing panels? Decision support? Clear instructions for procurement?
Confidentiality and privacy	HIPAA compliant and patient privacy protected at all interfaces Data integrity and security
Referring and reference laboratory information systems interface	Bidirectional? Automated? Manual elements? Critical value process?
Reference laboratory and EHR, ordering provider result interface	Will results go through the referring LIS? Will they be directly resulted into the EHR? Will they appear somewhere intuitive in the EHR? Results scanned in as an image? Results manually transcribed?
Formatting post-interface	Abnormal elements: asterisk, exclamation point, bold, color? Reference ranges correct? Alignment of results with headings?

Abbreviations: EHR, electronic health record; HIPAA, health insurance portability and accountability act; IT, information technology; LIS, laboratory information system.

management of low-volume, high-complexity tests performed offsite. The declining workforce in all parts of laboratory medicine create further challenges to adequate monitoring.[45,46] A schema of typical reference laboratory testing governance, oversight, and reporting relationships is laid out in **Fig. 5**.

All referring laboratories with a significant send-out volume should consider designating a medical director to review on a regular basis all processes, feedback, and metrics relevant to reference laboratories. This director should assemble a multidisciplinary

Table 5
Types of healthcare IT integration for reference laboratories and accompanying patient safety challenges

Systems and EHRs	Challenges
Print	Missed/lost results, report to wrong user
Fax	Missed/lost results, report to wrong user
Manual scanning into EHR	Report challenging to find in medical record, inability to trend results
Manual entry into EHR	Prone to clerical result transcription error
Direct interface	Result formatting with interpretative errors i.e, reference range appears under "result," loss of special formatting of critical/abnormal values, duplicate results, test tracking alarm fatigue for ordering providers

Abbreviation: EHR, electronic health record; IT, information technology.

Reference Laboratory Testing Governance and Oversight

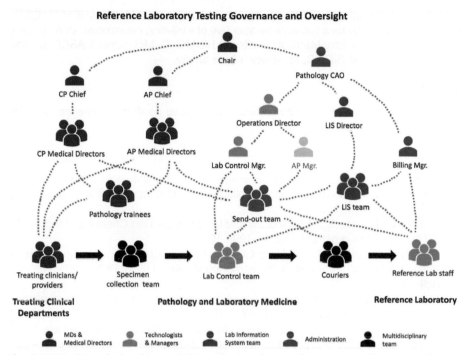

Fig. 5. Reporting relationships and hierarchy in reference laboratory testing oversight. AP, anatomic pathology; CAO, chief administrative officer; CP, clinical pathology; LIS, laboratory information system; MD, physician; Mgr, manager.

"send-outs" team, including managerial staff, treating clinicians, IT leaders, and legal, contracting, and billing experts. Both the medical director and the manager of the referring laboratory should have a clear counterpart in the reference laboratory leadership.

The need to ensure the quality and safety of reference laboratory testing, and the demands of CLIA '88, require that leaders resist the urge to say "we don't have control" of reference laboratories and thus "we are unable to improve quality." We must instead extend our oversight beyond what is under direct laboratory control, to ensure that in working with reference laboratories something's gained and nothing's lost.[47]

SUMMARY

Reference laboratories are critical to the delivery of pathology services and offer compelling clinical, operational, and economic benefits to the modern functioning laboratory. However, novel threats to patient safety and quality arise in referring-reference laboratory interactions and must be actively managed. Quality metrics, a safety checklist, thoughtful IT integration, feedback from clinical partners, and clear governance are all critical to reducing risk and improving safety when working with reference laboratories.

ACKNOWLEDGMENTS

Yigu Chen, Principal Associate at Harvard Medical School and Patient Safety Specialist at Beth Israel Deaconess Medical Center for his assistance with generating figures, Christopher Garniss (former laboratory medicine send-outs manager at

BIDMC and manager at Quest Diagnostics), neurologist Dr A. A. Beesen of St. Elizabeth's Medical Center for a valuable perspective of a treating neurologist, Dr A. Z. Herskovits, Clinical Chemistry Medical Director at BIDMC, G. McCormack ASCP, former operations director at BIDMC, for review of the article.

DISCLOSURE

The author does not have any commercial or financial conflicts of interest nor any funding sources to disclose.

REFERENCES

1. Weiss RL, Brown MS. Laboratory management and quality control. In: Jones SL, editor. Clinical laboratory pearls. Philadelphia: Lippincott Williams & Wilkins; 2001. p. 568–71.
2. Plebani M. The changing face of clinical laboratories. Clin Chem Lab Med 1999; 37(7). https://doi.org/10.1515/cclm.1999.109.
3. Plebani M, Laposata M, Lundberg GD. The brain-to-brain loop concept for laboratory testing 40 Years after its introduction. Am J Clin Pathol 2011;136(6): 829–33.
4. Plebani M. Charting the course of medical laboratories in a changing environment. Clin Chim Acta 2002;319(2):87–100.
5. Plebani M, Lippi G. Is laboratory medicine a dying profession? Blessed are those who have not seen and yet have believed. Clin Biochem 2010;43(12):939–41.
6. Plebani M. Clinical laboratory: factory or zero kilometer service? Clin Chim Acta 2020;503:228–30.
7. Lippi G, Guidi GC, Plebani M. One hundred years of laboratory testing and patient safety. Clin Chem Lab Med 2007;45(6):797–8.
8. Quest Diagnostics Products and Services. Quest diagnostics. Available at: https://www.questdiagnostics.com/home/about/products-services/. Accessed April 27, 2020.
9. Clinical Laboratory Improvement Amendments (CLIA). Regulations and guidance. Center for Medicare and Medicaid Services; 2020. Available at: https://www.cms.gov/Regulations-and-Guidance/Legislation/CLIA. Accessed May 1, 2020.
10. Ehrmeyer SS, Laessig RH. Regulatory requirements (CLIA '88, JCAHO, CAP) for decentralized testing. Am J Clin Pathol 1995;104(4 Suppl 1):S40–9.
11. Balogh E, Miller BT, Ball J. Improving diagnosis in health care. Washington, DC: The National Academies Press; 2015.
12. Norman GR, Eva KW. Diagnostic error and clinical reasoning. Med Educ 2010; 44(1):94–100.
13. Singh H, Graber ML. Improving diagnosis in health care — the next imperative for patient safety. N Engl J Med 2015;373(26):2493–5.
14. Plebani M. Laboratory-associated and diagnostic errors: a neglected link. Diagnosis 2014;1(1):89–94.
15. Graber ML, Plebani M. Diagnosis: a new era, a new journal. Diagnosis 2014; 1(1):1–2.
16. Khullar D, Jha AK, Jena AB. Reducing diagnostic errors — why now? N Engl J Med 2015;373(26):2491–3.
17. Graber ML. The physician and the laboratory: partners in reducing diagnostic error related to laboratory testing. Am J Clin Pathol 2006;126(Suppl 1):S44–7.

18. Plebani M. Exploring the iceberg of errors in laboratory medicine. Clin Chim Acta 2009;404(1):16–23.
19. Lippi G, Becan-Mcbride K, Behúlová D, et al. Preanalytical quality improvement: in quality we trust. Clin Chem Lab Med 2013;51(1):229–41.
20. Plebani M. The CCLM contribution to improvements in quality and patient safety. Clin Chem Lab Med 2013;51(1):39–46.
21. Sciacovelli L, Plebani M. The IFCC Working Group on laboratory errors and patient safety. Clin Chim Acta 2009;404(1):79–85.
22. Laposata M, Dighe A. "Pre-pre" and "post-post" analytical error: high-incidence patient safety hazards involving the clinical laboratory. Clin Chem Lab Med 2007;45(6):712–9.
23. Heher YK, Chen Y, Vanderlaan PA. Pre-analytic error: a significant patient safety risk. Cancer Cytopathol 2018;126(S8):738–44.
24. Heher YK, Chen Y, Vanderlaan PA. Measuring and assuring quality performance in cytology: a toolkit. Cancer Cytopathol 2017;125(S6):502–7.
25. Plebani M, Sciacovelli L, Marinova M, et al. Quality indicators in laboratory medicine: a fundamental tool for quality and patient safety. Clin Biochem 2013; 46(13–14):1170–4.
26. Heher YK. Elements of pathology dashboards. Vancouver, British Columbia, Canada: Association of Directors of Anatomic and Surgical Pathology; 2018. Available at: https://slideplayer.com/slide/14789376/. Accessed April 1, 2020.
27. Plebani M. The detection and prevention of errors in laboratory medicine. Ann Clin Biochem 2009;47(2):101–10.
28. Sciacovelli L, Lippi G, Sumarac Z, et al. Quality indicators in laboratory medicine: the status of the progress of IFCC working group "laboratory errors and patient safety" project. Clin Chem Lab Med 2017;55(3):348–57.
29. Vanderlaan PA, Chen Y, Distasio M, et al. Molecular testing turnaround time in non–small-cell lung cancer: monitoring a moving target. Clin Lung Cancer 2018;19(5):e589–90.
30. Gawande A. The checklist manifesto: how to get things right. London: Profile Books; 2011.
31. Chen Y, Anderson KR, Xu J, et al. Frozen-section checklist implementation improves quality and patient safety. Am J Clin Pathol 2019;151(6):607–12.
32. Higgins WY, Boorman DJ. An analysis of the effectiveness of checklists when combined with other processes, methods and tools to reduce risk in high hazard activities. Boeing Technical Journal 2016. Available at: https://www.boeing.com/resources/boeingdotcom/features/innovation-quarterly/2019_q3/BTJ_checklist_full.pdf. Accessed March 10, 2020.
33. Thomassen Ø, Espeland A, Søfteland E, et al. Implementation of checklists in health care; learning from high-reliability organisations. Scand J Trauma Resusc Emerg Med 2011;19(1):53. Available at: https://www.ncbi.nlm.nih.gov/pmc/articles/PMC7282392/.
34. Ely JW, Graber ML, Croskerry P. Checklists to reduce diagnostic errors. Acad Med 2011;86(3):307–13.
35. Plebani M. Errors in clinical laboratories or errors in laboratory medicine? Clin Chem Lab Med 2006;44(6):750–9.
36. Plebani M. Errors in laboratory medicine and patient safety: the road ahead. Clin Chem Lab Med 2007;45(6):700–7.
37. Plebani M, Ceriotti F, Messeri G, et al. Laboratory network of excellence: enhancing patient safety and service effectiveness. Clin Chem Lab Med 2006; 44(2):150–60.

38. Mate KS, Compton-Phillips AL. The antidote to fragmented health care. Harv Bus Rev 2014. Available at: https://hbr.org/2014/12/the-antidote-to-fragmented-health-care. Accessed May 10, 2020.

39. Edmonson AC. The kinds of teams health care needs. 2016. Available at: https://hbr.org/2015/12/the-kinds-of-teams-health-care-needs. Accessed May 10, 2020.

40. Bates DW, Singh H. Two decades since to err is human: an assessment of progress and emerging priorities in patient safety. Health Aff (Millwood) 2018;37(11): 1736–43.

41. Kay J. Technology to improve quality and accountability. Clin Chem Lab Med 2006;44(6):568–71.

42. Roy CL, Poon EG, Karson AS, et al. Patient safety concerns arising from test results that return after hospital discharge. Ann Intern Med 2005;143(2):121.

43. Meaningful use, electronic health record incentive programs and promoting interoperability (PI) programs. 2016 CMS program requirements. Center for Medicaid and Medicare Services; 2019. Available at: https://www.cms.gov/Regulations-and-Guidance/Legislation/EHRIncentivePrograms/2016ProgramRequirements. Accessed April 15, 2020.

44. Horowitz GL. The power of asterisks. Clin Chem 2015;61(8):1009–11.

45. Carden R, Allsbrook K, Thomas R. An examination of the supply and demand for clinical laboratory professionals in the United States. Transfusion 2009;49(11pt2): 2520–3.

46. The medical laboratory personnel shortage. American Society of Clinical Pathology. Available at: https://www.ascp.org/content/docs/default-source/policy-statements/ascp-pdft-pp-med-lab-personnel-short.pdf?sfvrsn=2. Accessed April 10, 2020.

47. Mitchell J. "Both Sides, now". Clouds, A&M Studios, May 1969, track 10. Available at: https://jonimitchell.com/music/album.cfm?id=3. Accessed March 30, 2020.

Diagnostic Testing for Patients with Spinal Muscular Atrophy

John F. Brandsema, MD[a,b],*, Brianna N. Gross, MS, LCGC[a],
Susan E. Matesanz, MD[a]

KEYWORDS

- Spinal muscular atrophy • Survival motor neuron • SMN1 • SMN2
- Newborn screening

KEY POINTS

- With new treatment options for spinal muscular atrophy, early and prompt diagnosis is key to ensuring best possible clinical outcomes.
- Newborn screening is an accurate tool to identify the vast majority of patients with spinal muscular atrophy.
- Carrier screening in women who are planning a pregnancy or who are currently pregnant will also contribute to early identification of patients with spinal muscular atrophy.
- Even with universal screening for homozygous *SMN1* deletion, approximately 5% of patients with spinal muscular atrophy would be missed because they are survival motor neuron deficient owing to compound heterozygosity and would continue to present symptomatically.
- Additional biomarkers to predict severity of spinal muscular atrophy phenotype are needed.

INTRODUCTION

Spinal muscular atrophy (SMA) is an autosomal recessive inherited disorder that leads to progressive muscular weakness owing to loss of alpha-motor neurons in the spinal cord and brainstem due to a mutation in the survival motor neuron 1 (*SMN1*) gene on chromosome 5q11.2 to 13.3. The incidence of the disease is estimated to be in 1 in 11,000.[1,2] Historically, the disease has been classified into 3 main types in childhood based on highest motor milestone achieved, with subtypes within each group

[a] Division of Neurology, Colket Translational Research Building, 10th Floor, 3501 Civic Center Boulevard, Philadelphia, PA 19104, USA; [b] Perelman School of Medicine, University of Pennsylvania, Philadelphia, PA, USA
* Corresponding author. Division of Neurology, Colket Translational Research Building, 10th Floor, 3501 Civic Center Boulevard Philadelphia, PA 19104.
E-mail address: brandsemaj@email.chop.edu

Clin Lab Med 40 (2020) 357–367
https://doi.org/10.1016/j.cll.2020.05.005
0272-2712/20/© 2020 Elsevier Inc. All rights reserved.
labmed.theclinics.com

(**Table 1**). A similar gene, *SMN2*, encodes a protein that only produces 10% to 15% of functional protein, with the rest of the protein produced rapidly degraded. *SMN2* copy number typically correlates with disease severity, with those with fewer copies of *SMN2* tending to have more severe disease (**Fig. 1**).[3,4] In the most severe form, type 1, which accounts for approximately 60% of all SMA, the majority of patients die by age 2 unless tube nutrition and mechanical ventilation are initiated.[5,6] With 2 new disease-modifying treatments approved by the US Food and Drug Administration available for SMA, prompt and accurate diagnosis of this disease is of critical importance. The newly available treatments, nusinersen approved in December 2016,[7] and onasemnogene abeparvovec-xioi approved in May 2019,[8] have led to alteration of the classically described phenotypes of disease.[9–12] Pivotal clinical trials have emphasized that early initiation of treatment leads to improved outcomes.[12–15] With disease-modifying treatments now available, prompt and rapid diagnosis of SMA is essential.

STRUCTURE OF *SMN1* AND *SMN2*

Within the 5q13 region, there are 2 highly homologous genes, *SMN1* and *SMN2*.[16] The 20-kB genes contain 9 exons, with a stop codon located near the end of exon 7, and produces a protein containing 294 amino acids.[17] The telomeric *SMN1* and centromeric *SMN2* genes are arranged in an inverted duplication. There are 5 single nucleotide differences between the *SMN1* and *SMN2*.[18] However, it is a single base pair difference (840C > T) in the coding regions between *SMN1* and *SMN2* (**Fig. 2**), which does not alter amino acid structure, but leads to alternative splicing and, thus, degradation of the majority of protein produced by *SMN2*.[17,19]

DIAGNOSIS OF SYMPTOMATIC PATIENTS

In untreated SMA, patients typically present with progressive skeletal muscle weakness and atrophy and absent deep tendon reflexes; the more severe forms also have progressive respiratory muscle weakness that relatively spares the diaphragm, and bulbar weakness leading to tongue fasciculations, dysarthria, and dysphagia.

More than 95% of patients with SMA will have a homozygous deletion of *SMN1*. The remaining 5% have pathogenic variants that will not be detected by deletion testing alone.[20] Owing to the Hardy-Weinberg equilibrium, the majority of these remaining patients will have a deletion in 1 allele and a point mutation (intragenic missense, nonsense, or frameshift variant) in *SMN1* on the other allele, leading to a compound heterozygote state.[19,20]

It is crucial to identify the methods used by the laboratory which is used for SMA testing. Laboratories commonly use multiplex ligation probe amplification (MLPA) methods to evaluate for deletions, real-time polymerase chain reaction (PCR) for deletions, or restriction fragment length polymorphism PCR to determine homozygous deletions.[21–26] If the patient is positive for SMA, these methods are then used to further evaluate *SMN2* copy number, except in the instance of homozygous deletion testing such as with PCR restriction fragment length polymorphism. It is important to identify whether a laboratory tests for deletions in the *SMN1* gene or if it will test for homozygous deletions. There is no consensus across laboratories on which method is best, and therefore physical examination, risk, and family history will be the best determining factor on which laboratory method should be selected for testing. These methods are highly accurate in determining a diagnosis of SMA. To capture the approximately 5% of patients who do not have homozygous deletions of *SMN1*, sequencing of the *SMN1* gene needs to be performed. Next-generation sequencing can be used to detect

Table 1
Clinical classification of SMA

MA Type	Other Names	Age at Onset	Life Span	Highest Motor Milestone Achieved	Other Features	Proportion of Total SMA (%)
Type IA	Prenatal, congenital SMA, Werdnig-Hoffman disease	Prenatal	<6 mo	Mostly unable to achieve motor milestones	Severe weakness at birth Profound hypotonia Facial diplegia Areflexia Early respiratory failure Joint contractures	60[a]
Type IB, type IC	Werdnig-Hoffman disease, Severe SMA ("non-sitters")	Type IB (0–3 mo) Type IC (3–6 mo)	<2 y without respiratory support	Never sits supported	Weakness "Frog leg" posture, hypotonia Tongue fasciculations Hyporeflexia, areflexia Suck and swallow difficulties Respiratory failure	60[a]
Type II	Intermediate SMA ("sitters"), Dubowitz disease	6–18 mo	>2 y ~ 70% alive at 25 y of age	Sits independently; never stands or walks	Proximal weakness, hypotonia Postural hand tremor Hyporeflexia Average or above average intellectual skills by adolescence Scoliosis	27
Type III	Kugelberg-Welander disease, mild SMA ("walkers")	>18 mo type IIIA (before 3 y) type IIIB (after 3 y)	Almost normal	Stands and walks	May have hand tremor Resembles muscular dystrophy	12
Type IV	Adult SMA	>21 y	Normal	Normal		1

[a] SMA types I, IA, IB, and IC all have a 60% proportion of total SMA.
Adapted from Markowitz JA, Singh P, Darras BT. Spinal muscular atrophy: a clinical and research update. Pediatr Neurol. 2016;46(1):2; with permission.

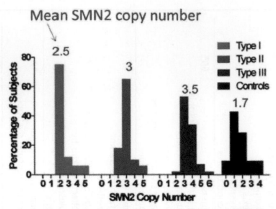

Fig. 1. SMN2 copy number in SMA and subject controls. (*Modified from* Crawford TO, Paushkin SV, Kobayashi DT, et al. Evaluation of SMN protein, transcript, and copy number in the biomarkers for spinal muscular atrophy (BforSMA) clinical study. PLoS One. 2012;7(4):e33572.)

sequence variants within genes, and has the ability to identify copy number variants of the SMN1 gene. Many laboratories will confirm via Sanger sequencing, although Sanger sequencing may be performed instead of next-generation sequencing, depending on the laboratory.[27,28] Sanger sequencing is considered the gold standard. Sequencing is a more complete test, in terms of capturing affected individuals; however, the turn-around time is lengthy. A difficulty with point mutations detected through sequencing is when a variant of uncertain significance is reported. This result may return because

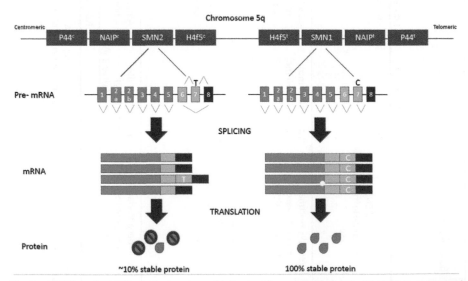

Fig. 2. *SMN1* and *SMN2* gene structure. (*Adapted from* Swoboda KJ. Of SMN in mice and men: a therapeutic opportunity. J Clin Invest. 2011;121(8):2980; with permission; and Butchbach MER. Copy number variations in the survival motor neuron genes: Implications for spinal muscular atrophy and other neurodegenerative diseases. Front Mol Biosci. 2016;3(MAR).)

laboratories may not be able to determine whether the point mutation is in *SMN1* or *SMN2* accurately, owing to the homology between the 2 genes, or because of the lack of other individuals with SMA and the same variant.[29] Clinical examination and determining if the sequence variant has been reported in other affected individuals will be crucial to making the diagnosis. Parental testing may provide further clarification if the deletion and sequence variant were identified to be inherited from a single parent and are therefore in cis.

NEWBORN SCREENING

In February of 2018, the US Food and Drug Administration voted to recommend that SMA be added to the recommended universal screening program in the United States.[30] As of September 2019, newborn screening has been adopted and implemented in 10 states, adopted but not yet implemented in 18 states, and piloted in 3 states.[31] It is estimated that universal adoption of NBS for SMA will identify 364 patients annually, 196 of whom will be type 1 patients. It is further estimated that such early identification will prevent approximately 50 patients from ventilator dependence and 30 deaths annually.[32] NBS currently only identifies homozygous deletions of *SMN1*, and therefore detects approximately 95% of Infants with SMA; consequently, it misses 5% of infants with SMA who have a heterozygous deletion and a pathogenic sequence variant.

A pilot study of NBS for SMA in New York state used dried blood spot (DBS) samples, and then a multiplex TaqMan real-time PCR assay validated to detect exon 7 deletions on both *SMN1* alleles.[33] Screening resulted in 1 suspected case, who was then confirmed for homozygous deletion and evaluated for *SMN2* copy number. A Taiwanese pilot study of NBS for SMA used an real-time PCR genotyping assay of *SMN1/SMN2* intron 7 to detect homozygous deletions in exon 7 of *SMN1* for first-tier screening. Second-tier screening used both droplet digital PCR from the same DBS sample, and multiplex ligation-dependent probe amplification from whole blood samples to confirm homozygous deletion and determine SMN2 copy number.[34]

Droplet digital PCR can be performed from DBS, whereas multiplex ligation-dependent probe amplification requires larger amounts of blood. Droplet digital PCR has been shown to extremely sensitive and specific for both detection of homozygous deletions in *SMN1*, *SMN2* copy number variation, and carrier status.[35] First tier screening for homozygous deletion in *SMN1* can be detected simultaneously from the same DBS punched used to test for severe combined immunodeficiency,[35,36] which allows for improved efficiency and easier implementation of screening.

Screening methods used have shown a 100% positive predictive value, with no reported false positives to date.[32] Whether or not to report carrier status remains an ongoing discussion. Estimated costs of adding SMA to existing NBS programs is $0.10 to $1.00, with the higher end of the range including second-tier screening to assess for *SMN2* copy number. The majority of state NBS programs estimated that it would take 1 to 3 years to implement NBS for SMA. Top identified challenges to implementation included ensuring availability and readiness of SMA specialists and ensuring sustainable support for SMA.[32]

Although procedures may vary slightly between states, generally, when a positive screen is identified, 2 points of contact are notified of the results. The laboratory identifies an NBS site that is closest in distance to the affected infant, where a designated contact at that institution is notified via the NBS portal and a phone call. The laboratory simultaneously will notify the pediatrician who was listed at the time of birth. The NBS site contact typically will reach out to the pediatrician to formulate a disclosure plan.

After the disclosure occurs, the family is brought to the NBS site for an evaluation, a detailed conversation about SMA, treatment plans, and confirmatory testing. Confirmatory testing can be sent to commercial laboratories, or to hospital in-house laboratories, based on the preference of the site. Many NBS laboratories will offer a repeat blood spot to reanalyze the sample to ensure there was no internal laboratory errors, such as switching of samples (**Fig. 3**).

CARRIER SCREENING AND PRENATAL DIAGNOSIS

In March of 2017, the American College of Obstetricians and Gynecologists recommended that SMA carrier screening should be offered to all women who are considering a pregnancy or who are already pregnant.[37] If a woman is found to be an SMA carrier, her partner should then be tested for carrier status; if a partner also tests positive, prenatal diagnosis can be offered.

Carrier testing is typically performed as part of a commercial panel that includes many other autosomal recessive inherited genetic disorders. In the United States, overall carrier frequency is estimated to be 1 in 54, and is highest among Caucasians[1] and lowest among Hispanic individuals[37,38] (**Table 2**). Each laboratory uses different methods to test for SMA carrier status. Most laboratories use next-generation sequencing to analyze the *SMN1* and *SMN2* genes, and many will use confirmatory methods such as Sanger sequencing and multiplex ligation-dependent probe amplification upon finding a pathogenic deletion or variant.[19,21,27,39] A large limitation to testing for carrier status is determining if the *SMN1* copies are in cis or are in trans. Silent carriers, or 2+0 carriers, comprise 3.7% of SMA carriers.[27] A silent carrier is an individual who has 2 *SMN1* copies in cis, and current technologies are unable to detect because it cannot identify the haplotype phase (**Fig. 4**). Therefore, the residual risk for carrier status is higher upon a negative carrier screen or a carrier screening result identifying 2 copies of *SMN1*.[39] *SMN1* copies in cis are more common among individuals of Ashkenazi Jewish descent and African descent.[38] One way to further lower the residual risk of carrier status is to test individuals for single nucleotide polymorphisms (SNP) that are known to co-occur when 2 SMN1 copies are in cis. The SNP that is looked at is *SMN1* c.*3 + 80T > G (g.27134 T > G).[40–42] This SNP is located in intron 7 of the SMN1 gene. There is a second SNP that can be looked at as well, c.*211_*212del (g.27706_27707delAT), which is located in exon 8.[42] Not all carrier screening tests provide information on the presence or absence of the SNPs.

Prenatal testing can be performed upon identification of carrier status of 2 parents, or if 1 parent is a carrier and the other parent has a higher residual risk to be a silent carrier. There are 2 ways to go about testing a pregnancy. Chorionic villus sampling can be performed at approximately 10 to 13 weeks of gestation. This method takes a sample of the chorionic villi, which is formed from the same cells from which the fetus is formed. The sample is then sent to a laboratory of choice to begin analysis of *SMN1* and *SMN2* genes. Amniocentesis can be performed at approximately 15 weeks of gestation and will take a sample of the amniotic fluid. The amniotic fluid contains cells

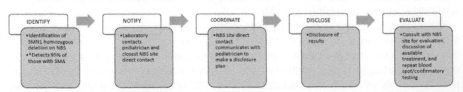

Fig. 3. Newborn screening process.

Table 2
Prior and adjusted risk for SMA carrier status when 2 or 3 *SMN1* copies are detected by quantitative assays

| Ethnicity | Prior Risk[a] | Adjusted Risk | |
		2 Copies	3 copies[b]
Caucasian	1:35	1:632	1:3500
Ashkenazi Jewish	1:41	1:350	1:4000
Asian	1:53	1:628	1:5000
African American	1:66	1:121	1:3000
Hispanic	1:117	1:1061	1:11,000

[a] Prior risk is the probability of having any carrier genotype $(1 + 0, 1+1^D, 2 + 0$ and $2+1^D)$.
[b] The risk estimates were rounded to 2 significant digits owing to approximations in their calculations.
From Hendrickson BC, Donohoe C, Akmaev VR, et al. Differences in SMN1 allele frequencies among ethnic groups within North America. J Med Genet. 2009;46(9):643; with permission.

from the fetus that are analyzed at the laboratory of choice for testing. Maternal contamination studies are performed for both chorionic villus sampling and amniocentesis to ensure that maternal cells did not contaminate the sample and that the results are representative of the fetus' genetic information.[43]

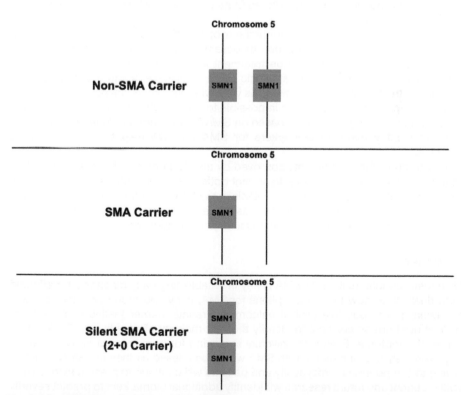

Fig. 4. Identification of silent carriers of SMA.

Preimplantation genetic testing for monogenic/single gene defects can be used before pregnancy if carrier parents are identified.[40] To perform preimplantation genetic testing for monogenic/single gene defects, in vitro fertilization must first occur. Methods for in vitro fertilization remain the same as it would for individuals with infertility struggles. Before the implantation procedure, embryos will have a few cells from the trophectoderm biopsied for genetic testing. Upon the completion of genetic testing, the SMN1 gene status is revealed for all embryos to select one for implantation into the uterus.[44–48]

TREATMENT OF SPINAL MUSCULAR ATROPHY

With the approval of 2 new treatments for SMA in recent years that can drastically alter the natural history of this disease, prompt identification of affected patients is critically important.

Early initiation of treatment is key in optimizing outcomes.[12–14] Nusinersen, an antisense oligonucleotide that upregulates SMN protein expression by SMN2 and is delivered via intrathecal injection in a dosing schedule that involves a 2-month loading phase followed by maintenance dosing every 4 months for life, is approved in patients of all ages with SMA. Onasemnogene abeparvovec-xioi gene therapy for SMA delivering self-promoting nonintegrating SMN to the nucleus of cells via a viral vector has initially only been approved for patients up to 2 years of age in an intravenous single-dose form. Accurate identification of SMN2 copy number is helpful in guiding treatment decisions for those with SMA. Expanding newborn screening to all states will allow families and clinicians in the United States to make the best treatment decisions for an individual patient.

For newborns with 2 or 3 copy numbers of SMN2, clear consensus exists that treatment should be initiated as soon as possible.[49] For those with 4 or more copy numbers of SMN2, the decision on treatment initiation is more nuanced. Because symptoms of SMA lag behind pathologic onset of disease, some argue for prompt initiation of treatment in these patients as well, whereas others advocate for a watchful waiting approach. Because it is impossible to predict when the exact onset of disease will occur in a given patient based on SMN2 copy number alone, work is being done to identify accurate biomarkers for SMA that will help to guide treatment decisions.

In addition to the 2 treatments approved by the US Food and Drug Administration that are available currently, other treatment options are being studied, and it is likely that additional medications will be available in the future. These include other genetic modulators of SMN protein expression, as well as phenotypic modulators that target augmenting nerve, muscle, or neuromuscular junction function.

SUMMARY

Diagnostic genetic testing for SMA is key in establishing early diagnosis for affected individuals. With new treatment options for SMA, early and prompt diagnosis is key to ensuring best possible clinical outcomes. Prenatal carrier testing of parents as well as newborn screening can identify the vast majority of people with SMA before onset of symptoms. Even with universal screening for homozygous SMN1 deletion, approximately 5% of patients with SMA would be missed as they are SMN deficient owing to compound heterozygosity and patients will continue to present symptomatically. Current and future research will identify additional biomarkers to predict severity of SMA phenotype as well as other treatment options.

REFERENCES

1. Sugarman EA, Nagan N, Zhu H, et al. Pan-ethnic carrier screening and prenatal diagnosis for spinal muscular atrophy: clinical laboratory analysis of >72 400 specimens. Eur J Hum Genet 2012;20(1):27–32.
2. Verhaart IEC, Robertson A, Wilson IJ, et al. Prevalence, incidence and carrier frequency of 5q-linked spinal muscular atrophy - a literature review. Orphanet J Rare Dis 2017;12(1).
3. Swoboda KJ, Prior TW, Scott CB, et al. Natural history of denervation in SMA: relation to age, SMN2 copy number, and function. Ann Neurol 2005. https://doi.org/10.1002/ana.20473.
4. Calucho M, Bernal S, Alías L, et al. Correlation between SMA type and SMN2 copy number revisited: an analysis of 625 unrelated Spanish patients and a compilation of 2834 reported cases. Neuromuscul Disord 2018. https://doi.org/10.1016/j.nmd.2018.01.003.
5. Finkel RS, McDermott MP, Kaufmann P, et al. Observational study of spinal muscular atrophy type I and implications for clinical trials. Neurology 2014; 83(9):810–7.
6. Kolb SJ, Coffey CS, Yankey JW, et al. Natural history of infantile-onset spinal muscular atrophy. Ann Neurol 2017;82(6):883–91.
7. Waldrop MA, Kolb SJ. Current treatment options in neurology—SMA therapeutics. Curr Treat Options Neurol 2019;21(6). https://doi.org/10.1007/s11940-019-0568-z.
8. FDA approves innovative gene therapy to treat pediatric patients with spinal muscular atrophy, a rare disease and leading genetic cause of infant mortality _ FDA. Available at: https://www.fda.gov/news-events/press-announcements/fda-approves-innovative-gene-therapy-treat-pediatric-patients-spinal-muscular-atrophy-rare-disease. Accessed October 14, 2019.
9. Finkel RS, Mercuri E, Darras BT, et al. Nusinersen versus sham control in infantile-onset spinal muscular atrophy. N Engl J Med 2017;377(18):1723–32.
10. Mercuri E, Darras BT, Chiriboga CA, et al. Nusinersen versus sham control in later-onset spinal muscular atrophy. N Engl J Med 2018;378(7):625–35.
11. Darras BT, Chiriboga CA, Iannaccone ST, et al. Nusinersen in later-onset spinal muscular atrophy: long-term results from the phase 1/2 studies. Neurology 2019;92(21):e2492–506.
12. Mendell JR, Al-Zaidy S, Shell R, et al. Single-dose gene-replacement therapy for spinal muscular atrophy. N Engl J Med 2017;377(18):1713–22.
13. Al-Zaidy SA, Mendell JR. From clinical trials to clinical practice: practical considerations for gene replacement therapy in SMA type 1. Pediatr Neurol 2019. https://doi.org/10.1016/j.pediatrneurol.2019.06.007.
14. De Vivo DC, Topaloglu H, Swoboda KJ, et al. Nusinersen in infants who initiate treatment in a presymptomatic stage of spinal muscular atrophy (SMA): interim efficacy and safety results from the phase 2 NURTURE study (S25.001). Neurology 2019;92(15 Supplement):S25–2001. Available at: http://n.neurology.org/content/92/15_Supplement/S25.001.abstract.
15. Darras BT, Markowitz JA, Monani UR, et al. Spinal muscular atrophies. In: Darras BT, Jones HR, Ryan MM, et al, editors. Neuromuscular disorders of infancy, childhood, and adolescence. 2nd edition. London: Elsevier/Academic Press; 2015. p. 117–45. Available at: https://www-clinicalkey-com.proxy.library.upenn.edu/#!/content/book/3-s2.0-B9780124170445000081. Accessed December 23, 2019.

16. Lefebvre S, Reboullet S, Clermont O, et al. Identification and characterization of a spinal muscular atrophy-determining gene. Cell 1995;80:155–65.

17. Bürglen L, Lefebvre S, Clermont O, et al. Structure and organization of the human survival motor neurone (SMN) gene. Genomics 1996;32(3):479–82.

18. Talbot K, Tizzano EF. The clinical landscape for SMA in a new therapeutic era. Gene Ther 2017;24(9):529–33.

19. Prior TW, Nagan N, Sugarman EA, et al. Technical standards and guidelines for spinal muscular atrophy testing. Genet Med 2011. https://doi.org/10.1097/GIM. 0b013e318220d523.

20. Wirth B. An update of the mutation spectrum of the survival motor neuron gene (SMN1) in autosomal recessive spinal muscular atrophy (SMA). Hum Mutat 2000;15:228–37.

21. Ogino S, Wilson RB. Spinal muscular atrophy: molecular genetics and diagnostics. Expert Rev Mol Diagn 2004;4:15–29.

22. Eijk-Van Os PGC, Schouten JP. Multiplex ligation-dependent probe amplification (MLPA ®) for the detection of copy number variation in genomic sequences. Methods Mol Biol 2011;688:97–126.

23. Rudnik-Schöneborn S, Eggermann T, Kress W, et al. Clinical utility gene card for: proximal spinal muscular atrophy. Eur J Hum Genet 2012;20(6):713.

24. Abbaszadegan MR, Keify F, Ashrafzadeh F, et al. Gene dosage analysis of proximal spinal muscular atrophy carriers using real-time PCR. Arch Iran Med 2011; 14(3):188–91.

25. Godinho FM de S, Bock H, Gheno TC, et al. Molecular analysis of spinal muscular atrophy: a genotyping protocol based on TaqMan® real-time PCR. Genet Mol Biol 2012;35(4 SUPPL):955–9.

26. van der Steege G, Grootscholten PM, van der Vlies P, et al. PCR-based DNA test to confirm clinical diagnosis of autosomal recessive spinal muscular atrophy. Lancet 1995;345(8955):985–6. Available at: http://www.ncbi.nlm.nih.gov/pubmed/7715313. Accessed December 16, 2019.

27. Feng Y, Ge X, Meng L, et al. The next generation of population-based spinal muscular atrophy carrier screening: comprehensive pan-ethnic SMN1 copy-number and sequence variant analysis by massively parallel sequencing. Genet Med 2017. https://doi.org/10.1038/gim.2016.215.

28. Yang L, Cao YY, Qu YJ, et al. [Sanger sequencing for the diagnosis of spinal muscular atrophy patients with survival motor neuron gene 1 compound heterozygous mutation]. Zhonghua Yi Xue Za Zhi 2017;97(6):418–23.

29. Richards S, Aziz N, Bale S, et al. Standards and guidelines for the interpretation of sequence variants: a joint consensus recommendation of the American College of medical genetics and Genomics and the Association for Molecular pathology. Genet Med 2015;17(5):405–24.

30. Health Bureau of the Health C. Newborn Screening for Spinal Muscular Atrophy A Summary of the Evidence and Advisory Committee Decision.; 2018. Available at: https://www.hrsa.gov/sites/default/files/hrsa/advisory-committees/heritable-dis orders/rusp/previous-nominations/sma-consumer-summary.pdf

31. Newborn screening for spinal muscular atrophy - Cure SMA. Available at: https:// www.curesma.org/newborn-screening-for-sma/. Accessed November 8, 2019.

32. Matern D, Tarini B, Kemper AR, et al. Evidence-based review of newborn screening for spinal muscular atrophy (SMA): final report (v5.2). Available at: https://www.hrsa.gov/sites/default/files/hrsa/advisory-committees/heritable-diso rders/reports-recommendations/sma-final-report.pdf. Accessed November 10, 2019.

33. Kraszewski JN, Kay DM, Stevens CF, et al. Pilot study of population-based newborn screening for spinal muscular atrophy in New York state. Genet Med 2017;20. https://doi.org/10.1038/gim.2017.152.

34. Chien Y-H, Chiang S-C, Weng W-C, et al. Presymptomatic diagnosis of spinal muscular atrophy through newborn screening. J Pediatr 2017;190. https://doi.org/10.1016/j.jpeds.2017.06.042.

35. Vidal-Folch N, Gavrilov D, Raymond K, et al. Multiplex droplet digital PCR method applicable to newborn screening, carrier status, and assessment of spinal muscular atrophy. Clin Chem 2018;64(12):1753–61.

36. Taylor JL, Lee FK, Yazdanpanah GK, et al. Newborn blood spot screening test using multiplexed real-time PCR to simultaneously screen for spinal muscular atrophy and severe combined immunodeficiency. Clin Chem 2015;61(2):412–9.

37. Romero S, Biggio JR, Saller DN, et al. Committee opinion: carrier screening for genetic Conditions. Vol 691. 2017. Available at: https://www.acog.org/-/media/Committee-Opinions/Committee-on-Genetics/co691.pdf?dmc=1&ts=20170224T0607157732. Accessed November 10, 2019.

38. Hendrickson BC, Donohoe C, Akmaev VR, et al. Differences in SMN1 allele frequencies among ethnic groups within North America. J Med Genet 2009;46(9):641–4.

39. Prior TW. Carrier screening for spinal muscular atrophy. Genet Med 2008;10(11):840–2.

40. Wu B. Introductory chapter: new theory and technology in early clinical embryogenesis. In: Bin Wu, Feng Huai L, editors. Embryology - theory and practice. London, UK: IntechOpen; 2019. https://doi.org/10.5772/intechopen.88331.

41. Alías L, Bernal S, Calucho M, et al. Utility of two SMN1 variants to improve spinal muscular atrophy carrier diagnosis and genetic counselling. Eur J Hum Genet 2018;26(10):1554–7.

42. Luo M, Liu L, Peter I, et al. An Ashkenazi Jewish SMN1 haplotype specific to duplication alleles improves pan-ethnic carrier screening for spinal muscular atrophy. Genet Med 2014;16(2):149–56.

43. Ghi T, Sotiriadis A, Calda P, et al. ISUOG practice guidelines: invasive procedures for prenatal diagnosis. Ultrasound Obstet Gynecol 2016;48(2):256–68.

44. De Rycke M, Goossens V, Kokkali G, et al. ESHRE PGD Consortium data collection XIV-XV: cycles from January 2011 to December 2012 with pregnancy follow-up to October 2013. Hum Reprod 2017;32(10):1974–94.

45. Parikh FR, Athalye AS, Naik NJ, et al. Preimplantation genetic testing: its evolution, where are we today? J Hum Reprod Sci 2018;11(4):306–14.

46. Sullivan-Pyke C, Dokras A. Preimplantation genetic screening and preimplantation genetic diagnosis. Obstet Gynecol Clin North Am 2018;45(1):113–25.

47. Lee VCY, Chow JFC, Yeung WSB, et al. Preimplantation genetic diagnosis for monogenic diseases. Best Pract Res Clin Obstet Gynaecol 2017;44:68–75.

48. Goldman KN, Nazem T, Berkeley A, et al. Preimplantation genetic diagnosis (PGD) for monogenic disorders: the value of concurrent aneuploidy screening. J Genet Couns 2016;25(6):1327–37.

49. Glascock J, Sampson J, Haidet-Phillips A, et al. Treatment algorithm for infants diagnosed with spinal muscular atrophy through newborn screening. J Neuromuscul Dis 2018;5(2):145–58.

Cerebrospinal Fluid Testing for Multiple Sclerosis

Joshua F. Goldsmith, DO, A. Zara Herskovits, MD, PhD*

KEYWORDS

- Multiple sclerosis • Cerebrospinal fluid • Isoelectric focusing • Biomarkers
- Autoimmune disease

KEY POINTS

- Laboratory analysis of cerebrospinal fluid to demonstrate intrathecal antibody synthesis can be used to inform clinical diagnosis and imaging studies for patients who are being evaluated for multiple sclerosis.
- Qualitative methods such as isoelectric focusing and quantitative techniques such as the immunoglobulin G index are commonly used methodologies for evaluating the production of intrathecal antibodies in cerebrospinal fluid.
- Measurement of kappa free light chains as well as markers of inflammation, axonal damage, and gliosis in cerebrospinal fluid are promising new approaches for the diagnosis of multiple sclerosis.

INTRODUCTION

Multiple sclerosis (MS) is one of the most common autoimmune diseases affecting the central nervous system (CNS). It is estimated that more than 2 million people worldwide have been diagnosed with this disorder and environmental, genetic, and epigenetic factors may contribute toward susceptibility.[1,2] The disease typically presents in young adults with one or more episodes of visual loss, diplopia, or other CNS dysfunction and these symptoms often spontaneously remit over the course of several weeks to months.[3] Some individuals experience a single event, termed Clinically Isolated Syndrome (CIS); however, most patients have a relapsing-remitting disease course over a period of 10 to 20 years.[3] MS often subsequently progresses into a secondary progressive phase characterized by more severe neurologic dysfunction. Roughly 10% of patients present with primary progressive MS, a disease subtype characterized by sustained, progressive neurologic symptoms.[3]

One of the major diagnostic challenges in MS is that clinical examination and imaging studies may vary substantially between and within patients over time.[4] Brain and

Department of Pathology, Beth Israel Deaconess Medical Center, 330 Brookline Avenue, Boston, MA 02215, USA
* Corresponding author.
E-mail address: aherskov@bidmc.harvard.edu

Clin Lab Med 40 (2020) 369–377
https://doi.org/10.1016/j.cll.2020.06.002
0272-2712/20/© 2020 Elsevier Inc. All rights reserved.

spinal cord MRI can be useful for detecting areas of demyelination, although these lesions have also been identified incidentally in patients who do not exhibit symptoms of MS.[5,6] Current guidelines characterize MS and related conditions based on clinical, imaging, and body fluid markers.[4]

Evaluation of cerebrospinal fluid (CSF) can be used to rule out inflammatory or infectious conditions in the differential diagnosis, and provides supporting evidence for MS by indicating that antibodies are intrathecally produced.[4] In this review, we describe the current practice of how CSF testing is performed and discuss new diagnostic approaches under development for MS.

INTRATHECAL ANTIBODY SYNTHESIS

For patients in whom MS is suspected, laboratory analysis of CSF to demonstrate intrathecal antibody synthesis maintains an important role in clinical diagnosis.[4,7] Several methods have been developed to analyze CSF for oligoclonal bands (OCBs) that are indicative of intrathecal antibody synthesis, including agarose gel electrophoresis (AGE), isoelectric focusing (IEF) and determination of the IgG index. Although the diagnostic sensitivity for MS varies depending on the analytical technique,[8–10] OCBs are detected in roughly 95% of patients with MS,[11] but can also be identified in many other conditions that can have neurologic manifestations including systemic lupus erythematosus, subacute sclerosing panencephalitis, or syphilis,[12] as well as in healthy controls.[13] For CIS, oligoclonal band detection is an independent risk factor in the development of a second attack.[7,14–18]

The gold standard for CSF diagnostic testing in MS is IEF, an electrophoretic technique that separates proteins along a pH gradient in a gel matrix, followed by immunoblotting to detect IgG oligoclonal bands. Alternative techniques include separation strategies that use agarose as the gel matrix to separate proteins by charge, or detection techniques that are nonspecific, such as silver staining, however these methods have reduced sensitivity and specificity relative to IEF.[19] Results from IEF can be interpreted qualitatively by evaluating matched serum and CSF samples drawn from the same patient. Oligoclonal bands present in the CSF that do not comigrate with bands in the serum sample are indicative of MS.[19]

Multiple studies over the past few decades have shown that IEF is a superior technique for detecting bands relative to high-resolution AGE.[20–23] Yet, according to the College of American Pathologists surveys, many laboratories have not adopted this technique, with only 61% of laboratories reporting the use of isoelectric focusing for oligoclonal band testing in 2019.[24] Some of the challenges that laboratories face in adopting IEF include the lack of methodological expertise, need for assay standardization, and interpretive variability.[10,25–27]

Both IEF and AGE assays represent qualitative approaches to demonstrating oligoclonal banding and the IgG index provides a quantitative method for providing further laboratory evidence of intrathecal antibody synthesis.[12] In this formula, the concentrations of albumin and IgG in both serum and CSF samples and the IgG index are expressed as a ratio (Equation 1).[28]

$$\text{IgG Index} = \frac{CSF\ IgG}{Serum\ IgG} \Big/ \frac{CSF\ Albumin}{Serum\ Albumin} \qquad \text{Equation 1}$$

Although it has been established that the IgG index correlates with the presence of oligoclonal bands in the CSF, studies show that this calculation has low diagnostic sensitivity, as some patients with a normal IgG index will still have oligoclonal bands by either AGE or IEF. The specificity of this test is also suboptimal, as some patients found to have an elevated IgG index may not ultimately have MS,[4,8,10,22] therefore the IgG index is best used in conjunction with qualitative methodologies such as IEF.

In addition to demonstrating intrathecal antibody synthesis, another important aspect of CSF testing is to rule out other conditions that may have an overlapping clinical presentation with MS. Neuromyelitis spectrum disorders (NMOSDs) are severe demyelinating conditions that predominantly target the optic nerves and spinal cord, although the brain and brainstem may also be involved. The clinical presentation of NMOSDs is similar to the early disease course of MS[4] and patients with both disorders can have OCBs in their CSF.[29] However, patients with NMOSD often develop Aquaporin-4 (AQP4)[4,30] autoantibodies that bind perivascular astrocytes, leading to complement activation and inflammation that cause oligodendrocyte damage and demyelination.[31] Some patients with NMOSDs who are seronegative for AQP4 develop antibodies against myelin oligodendrocyte glycoprotein (MOG), which is a component of myelin sheaths and oligodendrocyte membranes.[32]

Clinical guidelines recommend performing both AQP4 and MOG testing in patients with atypical presentations for MS that include bilateral optic neuritis or severe brainstem, spinal cord, or cerebral lesions. It is particularly important to rule out these conditions because some medications used to treat MS, such as interferon beta and natalizumab, can exacerbate NMOSD.[4]

CEREBROSPINAL FLUID DIAGNOSTICS UNDER DEVELOPMENT

Although the qualitative assessment of CSF oligoclonal IgG bands using isoelectric focusing is considered the gold standard to establish intrathecal synthesis of IgG,[33,34] its usage within clinical laboratories may be limited by lack of standardization and methodological expertise.[10,25,26] Therefore there is a need to develop robust, new diagnostic and prognostic tests for MS.

ANTIBODY-BASED CEREBROSPINAL FLUID DIAGNOSTICS

An emerging laboratory test that has garnered attention in recent years as a marker for MS is kappa free light chains (KFLCs) in CSF.[35] Although historically considered a T-cell–mediated disorder,[36] recent studies suggest that B cells and an expanded, clonal population of plasma cells play a role in the pathogenesis of MS.[37] In MS, plasma cell secretion of free light chains occurs in excess relative to the total amount of intact immunoglobulin. With this in mind, together with the introduction of new turbidimetric or nephelometric assays, investigators have turned their attention to evaluating quantitation of KFLC in CSF as a diagnostic tool in MS.[38,39]

Quantitative analysis of KFLCs in CSF is accomplished according to a multistep procedure. First, serum and CSF samples are obtained from patients with high clinical suspicion for MS and levels of albumin and KFLC levels are measured by nephelometry.[38] The ratio of CSF KFLCs to serum KFLCs is not used, as such a calculation lacks a reference to the blood-brain barrier.[40] Therefore, a separate calculation, referred to as the intrathecal fraction of KFLCs, is derived according to Equation 2, and is expressed as the KFLC index.[38,40,41]

$$\text{KFLC Index} = \frac{CSF\ KFLC}{Serum\ KFLC} \bigg/ \frac{CSF\ Albumin}{Serum\ Albumin} \qquad \text{Equation 2}$$

In a 2008 study by Presslauer and colleagues[41] in a study of 438 patients who underwent lumbar puncture, an empiric KFLC index value of greater than 5.9

was established as the level most suggestive of the diagnosis of MS. In this study, 67 of 70 patients with MS had a KFLC index greater than 5.9, which correlated with positive oligoclonal bands. Based on these data, the calculated diagnostic sensitivity for MS using KFLC index greater than 5.9 was 96%.[41] Although this study did not include a non-neurologic disease control group for comparison, as a proxy for healthy controls, a group of 45 patients under evaluation for normal pressure hydrocephalus, undefined dementia, or suspected but unconfirmed subarachnoid bleed and no clinical or subclinical evidence of inflammation was included. In these controls, the KFLC index was found to be 0.18, and the investigators suggested that this most likely would represent the KFLC index in a population of healthy controls.[41]

Since that time, more data have been published supporting the use of KFLC quantitation as a sensitive diagnostic tool in the evaluation of patients with MS. For example, a study published by Schwenkenbecher and colleagues[38] in 2018 implemented nephelometry to determine KFLCs in serum and CSF in 149 patients who experienced their first demyelinating event. They found an elevated KFLC index in 79 of 83 patients who were diagnosed with MS at baseline. Although the investigators concluded that detection of oligoclonal bands should retain its role in MS CSF diagnostic testing, it was suggested that KFLC index is a promising diagnostic technique to assess intrathecal immunoglobulin synthesis in multiple sclerosis, which could be used in addition to oligoclonal bands.[38]

Using a similar approach to the calculation of IgG synthesis, another related antibody parameter used as a biomarker is the quantification of intrathecally produced IgM in the CSF from patients with MS.[42,43] Several studies indicate that the production of intrathecal IgM may be associated with a worse prognosis,[44,45] and this parameter may be useful for predicting the conversion from CIS to MS.[43] Further investigations in large patient cohorts composed of different MS subtypes are needed to verify the clinical utility of measuring IgM and KFLC, but the existing literature suggests that these antibody-based CSF markers are extremely promising for diagnosis and prognosis of MS.

INFLAMMATORY MARKERS

Evaluating disease activity in MS is currently based primarily on clinical and MRI findings.[46] Predicting patients at risk for developing MS remains an elusive but important goal, and the development of CSF tests that allow clinicians to identify patients with subclinical disease are needed.[47] The role of cytokines and chemokines in the inflammatory response has been well established and their detection may allow clinicians to monitor disease activity in patients.[48] Associations between MS activity and CSF levels of the proinflammatory cytokines tumor necrosis factor-α and interleukin-6 have been described, although study results are mixed.[25,49–51]

Another promising CSF biomarker used to measure disease activity and progressive axonal degeneration is the chemokine ligand 13 (CXCL13), a B-cell chemoattractant that aids in the formation of B-cell follicles, a known component of MS pathogenesis.[47] For example, a study in 2013 found that for patients with secondary progressive and relapsing-remitting MS, levels of CXCL13 continuously increased over a period of 12 months, suggesting CXCL13 levels in CSF may correlate with disease progression in this cohort; however, more studies are needed, as data do not show clearly consistently reproducible results.[47,52] Ultimately, larger prospective studies evaluating the role of CXCL13 in the diagnosis of MS are needed.[47,53,54]

MARKERS OF AXONAL DAMAGE AND GLIOSIS

Other CSF markers that reflect disease activity, progression, and response to therapy in MS include neurofilament proteins, YKL-40 (also named Chitinase 3-Like 1 or CHI3L1) and glial fibrillary acidic protein (GFAP). However, similar to the inflammatory protein biomarkers, these analytes are not specific for MS when measured in the CSF because axonal damage and gliosis are processes common to many neurodegenerative conditions.

Neurofilaments are cytoskeletal proteins that are disrupted during axonal degeneration. Some of their components, particularly light chains, have been associated with gadolinium-enhancing MRI lesions, suggesting they may allow for disease screening.[55–57] Neurofilament light chains may also predict disease progression, and one study found that higher levels of neurofilament light chains in the CSF in early MS predict a higher multiple sclerosis severity score and a shorter time to conversion to secondary progressive MS after a median of 14 years of follow-up.[58]

YKL-40 is a glycoprotein expressed on microglia, macrophages, astrocytes, and epithelial cells. CSF levels of YKL-40 correlate with disease activity and are increased in patients with more rapid disease progression from CIS to MS.[59] High levels of YKL-40 and GFAP in the CSF at the time of diagnosis have also been linked with cognitive impairment and further longitudinal studies are required to examine this association.[60]

GFAP is a cytoskeletal protein found in astrocyte intermediate filaments that is elevated in the CSF of patients with MS, reflecting ongoing CNS injury. Further, it is suggested that CSF GFAP levels vary within patients with MS, with lower levels reflecting less severe disease and higher levels reflecting greater disease severity. These data and other studies indicate that laboratory evaluation of CSF GFAP may be of diagnostic and prognostic value.[61–63]

SUMMARY AND FUTURE DIRECTIONS

A variety of methods are currently used to analyze the CSF in patients with MS and many novel approaches are under investigation. As described herein, some of these, particularly kappa light chain levels, may provide sensitive and cost-effective diagnostic testing options that are not subjectively interpreted and can be performed with a rapid turnaround time using automated analyzers that are commonly used in a hospital laboratory.

The analysis of CSF plays an integral role in the diagnosis of MS. Although we have focused our discussion around current practice and a limited number of biomarkers with strong clinical evidence, there are many other technical approaches and target analytes currently under investigation. As further investigations in large patient cohorts composed of different MS subtypes validate the clinical utility of these tests, it seems likely that some of these markers may be incorporated into professional society guidelines in the future. Monitoring disease activity, progression, and response to therapy are important aspects of clinical management, and investigators are increasingly turning their attention toward potential biomarkers that can be used to guide therapeutic management for patients with MS.[47,64]

ACKNOWLEDGMENTS

The authors thank Dr Ursela Baber for her helpful review of this article.

DISCLOSURE

The authors have no funding sources that represent commercial or financial conflicts of interest.

REFERENCES

1. Wallin MT, Culpepper WJ, Nichols E, et al. Global, regional, and national burden of multiple sclerosis 1990–2016: a systematic analysis for the Global Burden of Disease Study 2016. Lancet Neurol 2019;18(3):269–85.
2. Thompson AJ, Baranzini SE, Geurts J, et al. Multiple sclerosis. Lancet 2018; 391(10130):1622–36.
3. Olek MJ, Howard J. Clinical presentation, course, and prognosis of multiple sclerosis in adults. Available at: https://www.uptodate.com/contents/clinical-presentation-course-and-prognosis-of-multiple-sclerosis-in-adults?search=multiple sclerosis&source=search_result&selectedTitle=1 ~ 150&usage_type=default& display_rank=1. Accessed March 11, 2020.
4. Thompson AJ, Banwell BL, Barkhof F, et al. Diagnosis of multiple sclerosis: 2017 revisions of the McDonald criteria. Lancet Neurol 2018;17(2):162–73.
5. Okuda D, Mowry E, Beheshtian A, et al. Incidental MRI anomalies suggestive of multiple sclerosis: the radiologically isolated syndrome. Neurology 2009;73(20): 1714.
6. Lebrun C, Kantarci OH, Siva A, et al. Anomalies characteristic of central nervous system demyelination: radiologically isolated syndrome. Neurol Clin 2018;36(1): 59–68.
7. Arrambide G, Tintore M. CSF examination still has value in the diagnosis of MS - Commentary. Mult Scler 2016. https://doi.org/10.1177/1352458516642033.
8. Andersson M, Alvarez-Cermeño J, Bernardi G, et al. Cerebrospinal fluid in the diagnosis of multiple sclerosis: a consensus report. J Neurol Neurosurg Psychiatry 1994. https://doi.org/10.1136/jnnp.57.8.897.
9. Stangel M, Fredrikson S, Meinl E, et al. The utility of cerebrospinal fluid analysis in patients with multiple sclerosis. Nat Rev Neurol 2013. https://doi.org/10.1038/nrneurol.2013.41.
10. Freedman MS, Thompson EJ, Deisenhammer F, et al. Recommended standard of cerebrospinal fluid analysis in the diagnosis of multiple sclerosis: a consensus statement. Arch Neurol 2005;62(6):865–70.
11. Deisenhammer F, Zetterberg H, Fitzner B, et al. The cerebrospinal fluid in multiple sclerosis. Front Immunol 2019;10:1–10.
12. Giovanni G. Cerebrospinal Fluid Analysis in Multiple Sclerosis and Related Disorders. Handbook of Clinical Neurology. (D.S. Goodin, Editor) Elsevier B.V.: Amsterdam, The Netherlands, 2014;122: 681-702. http://doi.org/10.1016/B978-0-444-52001-2.00029-7
13. Lo Sasso B, Agnello L, Bivona G, et al. Cerebrospinal fluid analysis in multiple sclerosis diagnosis: an update. Med 2019;55(6):3–7.
14. Tintoré M, Rovira A, Río J, et al. Do oligoclonal bands add information to MRI in first attacks of multiple sclerosis? Neurology 2008. https://doi.org/10.1212/01.wnl. 0000280576.73609.c6.
15. Dobson R, Ramagopalan S, Davis A, et al. Cerebrospinal fluid oligoclonal bands in multiple sclerosis and clinically isolated syndromes: a meta-analysis of prevalence, prognosis and effect of latitude. J Neurol Neurosurg Psychiatry 2013. https://doi.org/10.1136/jnnp-2012-304695.

16. Kuhle J, Disanto G, Dobson R, et al. Conversion from clinically isolated syndrome to multiple sclerosis: a large multicantre study. Mult Scler 2015. https://doi.org/10.1177/1352458514568827.

17. Tintore M, Rovira À, Río J, et al. Defining high, medium and low impact prognostic factors for developing multiple sclerosis. Brain 2015. https://doi.org/10.1093/brain/awv105.

18. Huss AM, Halbgebauer S, Öckl P, et al. Importance of cerebrospinal fluid analysis in the era of McDonald 2010 criteria. J Neurol 2016. https://doi.org/10.1007/s00415-016-8302-1.

19. Freedman MS, Thompson EJ, Deisenhammer F, et al. Cerebrospinal fluid analysis in the diagnosis of multiple sclerosis. Adv Neurol 2006;98:147–60.

20. Keren DF. Protein electrophoresis in clinical diagnosis. Chicago, Illinois: American Society for Clinical Pathology Press; 2012.

21. Fortini AS, Sanders EL, Weinshenker BG, et al. Cerebrospinal fluid oligoclonal bands in the diagnosis of multiple sclerosis: isoelectric focusing with IgG immunoblotting compared with high-resolution agarose gel electrophoresis and cerebrospinal fluid IgG index. Am J Clin Pathol 2003;120(5):672–5.

22. Lunding J, Midgard R, Vedeler CA. Oligoclonal bands in cerebrospinal fluid: a comparative study of isoelectric focusing, agarose gel electrophoresis and IgG index. Acta Neurol Scand 2000;102(5):322–5.

23. Peter JB, McKeown KL, Agopian MS. Assessment of different methods to detect increased autochthonous production of immunoglobulin G and oligoclonal immunoglobulins in multiple sclerosis. Am J Clin Pathol 1992;97(6):858–60.

24. College of American Pathologists. Cerebrospinal fluid chemistry and oligoclonal bands (M-B 2019). 2019.

25. Franciotta DM, Grimaldi LME, Martino GV, et al. Tumor necrosis factor in serum and cerebrospinal fluid of patients with multiple sclerosis. Ann Neurol 1989;26(6):787–9.

26. Ohman S, Ernerudh J, Forsberg P, et al. Comparison of seven formulae and isoelectrofocusing for determination of intrathecally produced IgG in neurological diseases. Ann Clin Biochem 1992;29(4):405–10.

27. Magliozzi R, Cross AH. Can CSF biomarkers predict future MS disease activity and severity? Mult Scler J 2020;26(5):582–90.

28. Link H, Tibbling G. Principles of albumin and IgG analyses in neurological disorders. III. evaluation of igg synthesis within the central nervous system in multiple sclerosis. Scand J Clin Lab Invest 1977;37(5):397–401.

29. Petzold A. Intrathecal oligoclonal IgG synthesis in multiple sclerosis. J Neuroimmunol 2013;262(1–2):1–10.

30. Papadopoulos MC, Bennett JL, Verkman AS. Treatment of neuromyelitis optica: state-of-the-art and emerging therapies. Nat Rev Neurol 2014. https://doi.org/10.1038/nrneurol.2014.141.

31. Papadopoulos MC, Verkman AS. Aquaporin 4 and neuromyelitis optica. Lancet Neurol 2012. https://doi.org/10.1016/S1474-4422(12)70133-3.

32. Di Pauli F, Berger T. Myelin oligodendrocyte glycoprotein antibody-associated disorders: toward a new spectrum of inflammatory demyelinating CNS disorders? Front Immunol 2018;9:1–12.

33. Menéndez-Valladares P, García-Sánchez M, Cuadri Benítez P, et al. Free kappa light chains in cerebrospinal fluid as a biomarker to assess risk conversion to multiple sclerosis. Mult Scler J Exp Transl Clin 2015;1. 205521731562093.

34. Bourahoui A, De Seze J, Guttierez R, et al. CSF isoelectrofocusing in a large cohort of MS and other neurological diseases. Eur J Neurol 2004;11(8):525–9.

35. Agnello L, Lo Sasso B, Salemi G, et al. Clinical use of κ free light chains index as a screening test for multiple sclerosis. Lab Med 2020. https://doi.org/10.1093/labmed/lmz073.

36. Zozulya AL, Wiendl H. The role of regulatory T cells in multiple sclerosis. Nat Clin Pract Neurol 2008;4:384–98.

37. Lehmann-Horn K, Kinzel S, Weber MS. Deciphering the role of B cells in multiple sclerosis—towards specific targeting of pathogenic function. Int J Mol Sci 2017; 18(10). https://doi.org/10.3390/ijms18102048.

38. Schwenkenbecher P, Konen FF, Wurster U, et al. The persisting significance of oligoclonal bands in the dawning era of kappa free light chains for the diagnosis of multiple sclerosis. Int J Mol Sci 2018;19(12). https://doi.org/10.3390/ijms19123796.

39. Bracco F, Gallo P, Menna R, et al. Free light chains in the CSF in multiple sclerosis. J Neurol 1987. https://doi.org/10.1007/BF00314285.

40. Presslauer S, Milosavljevic D, Huebl W, et al. Validation of kappa free light chains as a diagnostic biomarker in multiple sclerosis and clinically isolated syndrome: a multicenter study. Mult Scler 2016;22(4):502–10.

41. Presslauer S, Milosavljevic D, Brücke T, et al. Elevated levels of kappa free light chains in CSF support the diagnosis of multiple sclerosis. J Neurol 2008;255(10): 1508–14.

42. Forsberg P, Henriksson A, Link H, et al. Reference values for CSF-igm, CSF-igm/s-igm ratio and igm index, and its application to patients with multiple sclerosis and aseptic meningoencephalitis. Scand J Clin Lab Invest 1984;44(1):7–12.

43. Pfuhl C, Grittner U, Gieß RM, et al. Intrathecal IgM production is a strong risk factor for early conversion to multiple sclerosis. Neurology 2019;93(15):e1439–51.

44. Villar LM, Masjuan J, González-Porqué P, et al. Intrathecal IgM synthesis predicts the onset of new relapses and a worse disease course in MS. Neurology 2002; 59(4):555–9.

45. Perini P, Ranzato F, Calabrese M, et al. Intrathecal IgM production at clinical onset correlates with a more severe disease course in multiple sclerosis. J Neurol Neurosurg Psychiatry 2006;77(8):953–5.

46. Rotstein DL, Healy BC, Malik MT, et al. Evaluation of no evidence of disease activity in a 7-year longitudinal multiple sclerosis cohort. JAMA Neurol 2015;72(2): 152–8.

47. Domingues RB, Fernandes GBP, Leite FBV de M, et al. The cerebrospinal fluid in multiple sclerosis: far beyond the bands. Einstein (Sao Paulo). 2017;15(1):100–4.

48. Dendrou CA, Fugger L, Friese MA. Immunopathology of multiple sclerosis. Nat Rev Immunol 2015;15:545–58.

49. Vladić A, Horvat G, Vukadin S, et al. Cerebrospinal fluid and serum protein levels of tumour necrosis factor-alpha (TNF-α), interleukin-6 (IL-6) and soluble interleukin-6 receptor (sIL-6R gp80) in multiple sclerosis patients. Cytokine 2002;20(2):86–8.

50. Malmeström C, Andersson BA, Haghighi S, et al. IL-6 and CCL2 levels in CSF are associated with the clinical course of MS: implications for their possible immunopathogenic roles. J Neuroimmunol 2006;175(1–2):176–82.

51. Matsushita T, Tateishi T, Isobe N, et al. Characteristic cerebrospinal fluid cytokine/chemokine profiles in neuromyelitis optica, relapsing remitting or primary progressive multiple sclerosis. PLoS One 2013;8(4). https://doi.org/10.1371/journal.pone.0061835.

52. Romme Christensen J, Börnsen L, Khademi M, et al. CSF inflammation and axonal damage are increased and correlate in progressive multiple sclerosis. Mult Scler J 2013;19(7):877–84.
53. Alvarez E, Piccio L, Mikesell RJ, et al. CXCL13 is a biomarker of inflammation in multiple sclerosis, neuromyelitis optica, and other neurological conditions. Mult Scler J 2013;19(9):1204–8.
54. Ferraro D, Galli V, Vitetta F, et al. Cerebrospinal fluid CXCL13 in clinically isolated syndrome patients: association with oligoclonal IgM bands and prediction of multiple sclerosis diagnosis. J Neuroimmunol 2015. https://doi.org/10.1016/j.jneuroim.2015.04.011.
55. Gaiottino J, Norgren N, Dobson R, et al. Increased neurofilament light chain blood levels in neurodegenerative neurological diseases. PLoS One 2013;8(9). https://doi.org/10.1371/journal.pone.0075091.
56. Lycke JN, Karlsson JE, Andersen O, et al. Neurofilament protein in cerebrospinal fluid: a potential marker of activity in multiple sclerosis. J Neurol Neurosurg Psychiatry 1998;64(3):402–4.
57. Burman J, Zetterberg H, Fransson M, et al. Assessing tissue damage in multiple sclerosis: a biomarker approach. Acta Neurol Scand 2014;130(2):81–9.
58. Salzer J, Svenningsson A, Sundström P. Neurofilament light as a prognostic marker in multiple sclerosis. Mult Scler 2010;16(3):287–92.
59. Novakova L, Axelsson M, Khademi M, et al. Cerebrospinal fluid biomarkers as a measure of disease activity and treatment efficacy in relapsing-remitting multiple sclerosis. J Neurochem 2017;141(2):296–304.
60. Quintana E, Coll C, Salavedra-Pont J, et al. Cognitive impairment in early stages of multiple sclerosis is associated with high cerebrospinal fluid levels of chitinase 3-like 1 and neurofilament light chain. Eur J Neurol 2018;25(9):1189–91.
61. Rosengren LE, Lycke J, Andersen O. Glial fibrillary acidic protein in CSF of multiple sclerosis patients: relation to neurological deficit. J Neurol Sci 1995; 133(1–2):61–5.
62. Petzold A, Eikelenboom MJ, Gveric D, et al. Markers for different glial cell responses in multiple sclerosis: clinical and pathological correlations. Brain 2002; 125(7):1462–73.
63. Malmeström C, Haghighi S, Rosengren L, et al. Neurofilament light protein and glial fibrillary acidic protein as biological markers in MS. Neurology 2003. https://doi.org/10.1212/01.WNL.0000098880.19793.B6.
64. Salzer J. The only certain measure of the effectiveness of multiple sclerosis therapy is cerebrospinal neurofilament level - YES. Mult Scler 2015;21(10): 1239–40.

Moving?

Make sure your subscription moves with you!

To notify us of your new address, find your **Clinics Account Number** (located on your mailing label above your name), and contact customer service at:

Email: journalscustomerservice-usa@elsevier.com

800-654-2452 (subscribers in the U.S. & Canada)
314-447-8871 (subscribers outside of the U.S. & Canada)

Fax number: 314-447-8029

Elsevier Health Sciences Division
Subscription Customer Service
3251 Riverport Lane
Maryland Heights, MO 63043

*To ensure uninterrupted delivery of your subscription, please notify us at least 4 weeks in advance of move.

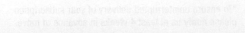

Printed and bound by CPI Group (UK) Ltd, Croydon, CR0 4YY

03/10/2024

01040480-0015